Medical Image Segmentation Using Level Set Method and Digital Topology

Xiao Han

Medical Image Segmentation Using Level Set Method and Digital Topology

Concepts and New Developments

VDM Verlag Dr. Müller

Impressum/Imprint (nur für Deutschland/ only for Germany)

Bibliografische Information der Deutschen Nationalbibliothek: Die Deutsche Nationalbibliothek verzeichnet diese Publikation in der Deutschen Nationalbibliografie; detaillierte bibliografische Daten sind im Internet über http://dnb.d-nb.de abrufbar.
Alle in diesem Buch genannten Marken und Produktnamen unterliegen warenzeichen-, marken- oder patentrechtlichem Schutz bzw. sind Warenzeichen oder eingetragene Warenzeichen der jeweiligen Inhaber. Die Wiedergabe von Marken, Produktnamen, Gebrauchsnamen, Handelsnamen, Warenbezeichnungen u.s.w. in diesem Werk berechtigt auch ohne besondere Kennzeichnung nicht zu der Annahme, dass solche Namen im Sinne der Warenzeichen- und Markenschutzgesetzgebung als frei zu betrachten wären und daher von jedermann benutzt werden dürften.

Coverbild: www.purestockx.com

Verlag: VDM Verlag Dr. Müller Aktiengesellschaft & Co. KG
Dudweiler Landstr. 99, 66123 Saarbrücken, Deutschland
Telefon +49 681 9100-698, Telefax +49 681 9100-988, Email: info@vdm-verlag.de
Zugl.: Baltimore, Johns Hopkins University, Diss., 2003

Herstellung in Deutschland:
Schaltungsdienst Lange o.H.G., Berlin
Books on Demand GmbH, Norderstedt
Reha GmbH, Saarbrücken
Amazon Distribution GmbH, Leipzig
ISBN: 978-3-639-11118-7

Imprint (only for USA, GB)

Bibliographic information published by the Deutsche Nationalbibliothek: The Deutsche Nationalbibliothek lists this publication in the Deutsche Nationalbibliografie; detailed bibliographic data are available in the Internet at http://dnb.d-nb.de.
Any brand names and product names mentioned in this book are subject to trademark, brand or patent protection and are trademarks or registered trademarks of their respective holders. The use of brand names, product names, common names, trade names, product descriptions etc. even without a particular marking in this works is in no way to be construed to mean that such names may be regarded as unrestricted in respect of trademark and brand protection legislation and could thus be used by anyone.

Cover image: www.purestockx.com

Publisher:
VDM Verlag Dr. Müller Aktiengesellschaft & Co. KG
Dudweiler Landstr. 99, 66123 Saarbrücken, Germany
Phone +49 681 9100-698, Fax +49 681 9100-988, Email: info@vdm-publishing.com

Printed in the U.S.A.
Printed in the U.K. by (see last page)
ISBN: 978-3-639-11118-7

Contents

1

Chapter 1

Introduction

1.1 Motivation

There have been dramatic advances in medical imaging technology over the past two decades. The advent of various methods such as magnetic resonance imaging (MRI), computed tomography (CT), magnetoencephalography (MEG), 3D ultrasound imaging, positron emission tomography (PET), single photon emission computed tomography (SPECT), and functional MRI (fMRI) has provided physicians with powerful, non-invasive ways for studying the internal anatomical structures and physiological processes of the human body [3]. The advances in imaging techniques also bring the benefit of providing better diagnosis and treatment options to a family of clinical applications. However, our ability to acquire images outstrips our ability to effectively analyze and interpret them. While it is now routine to gather full three-dimensional (3D) digital image data of the anatomy, experts cannot easily visualize the entire volume in 3D or always make reliable quantitative assessment of pathology or illness directly based on the raw data. To facilitate visualization, manipulation, and especially quantitative analysis of medical images, methods are needed for the repeatable, accurate and efficient localization and delineation of objects of interest from given multi-dimensional medical images. This object localization and delineation process is commonly referred to as image segmentation.

Approaches to image segmentation can be broadly classified as manual, semiautomatic, and automatic. Manual segmentation by experts is a tedious, difficult, and time consuming task, and is prone to error, bias, and poor reproducibility (inter- and intra-rater variabilities). For example, a high degree (up to 15%) of variance was reported when studying the segmentation consistency and reproducibility of human experts in segmenting brain cortical gray matter and brain tumors [4]. Semi-automatic or interactive segmentation can only partially eliminate these problems. It remains a prohibitive task to segment a large number of image data sets as is typically needed to get statistically significant results. Besides, both manual and interactive segmentations are usually limited to two-dimensional (2D) slice-wise processing due to the lack of suitable volume visualization tools. Such slice-by-slice segmentation suffers from difficulties in maintaining consistency across slices. The goal of this doctoral research was to develop generally applicable segmentation algorithms that can aid in the automation of medical image analysis tasks. Our driving application is the automatic, geometrically accurate, topologically correct, and reproducible reconstruction of the cortical surfaces from 3D MR images of human brains.

1.2 Tissue Segmentation and Cortical Surface Reconstruction from MR brain images

1.2.1 MR images of human brain

The brain is considered to be the most complex and yet least understood organ of the human body. The advent of magnetic resonance imaging (MRI) enables neuroscientists to look inside the brain in a non-invasive manner, providing valuable *in vivo* information about the brain structure for a wide variety of neuroscience and clinical purposes. Before we discuss the processing of MR brain images, we first summarize the basic principles of this imaging technique.

MRI has replaced CT as the best structural neuroimaging technique due to its unparalleled soft tissue contrast, high spatial resolution, and flexibility in the differentiation of various internal brain tissue classes. The principles of MR imaging can

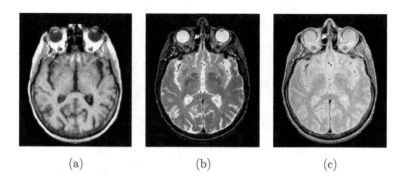

(a)　　　　　　　　　(b)　　　　　　　　　(c)

Figure 1.1: 2D slices of three types of MR images of the same brain: (a) a T1-weighted image slice, (b) a T2-weighted image slice, and (c) a PD-weighted image slice.

be found in [5]. Basically, the construction of an MR image relies on the resonance property of some nuclei present in the human body, in particular the hydrogen nuclei (the protons) of the water molecule. In a MRI scanner, the object is placed in a strong static magnetic field (1.5 Tesla, usually), which aligns the magnetic moments of individual protons. Sequences of radio-frequency (RF) excitation signals (known as *pulse sequences*) are then applied to excite the tissue to be imaged by tipping the net magnetic moment from its equilibrium position. During the relaxation of protons to their equilibrium state, an RF signal that encodes the position of the protons is generated. This RF signal, received by a receiver coil, produces the MR image after a reconstruction step that involves an inverse Fourier transform.

It is well known that the relaxation time constants (T1 for the *longitudinal relaxation time* and T2 for the *transverse relaxation time*) and the proton density (PD) differ in different tissue classes. Different pulse sequences can thus be designed to control the relative "weight" of these parameters to get different image contrast between the tissue classes, which generates the so called T1-, T2-, or PD-weighted MR images. One example is shown in Fig. 1.1, where the same brain has a different appearance when imaged with different pulse sequences. Overall, T1-weighted images have the best contrast across all (three) brain tissue classes and provide good anatomical details. Thus, they are used as the image source for our research on cortical surface

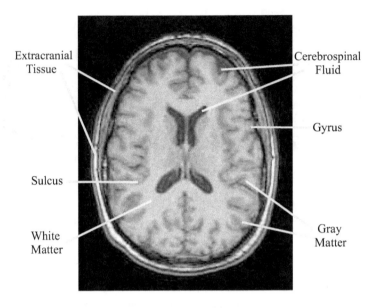

Figure 1.2: Cross-section of a T1-weighted MR image of the human brain.

reconstruction.

Fig. 1.2 shows a cross-section of another T1-weighted MR brain image volume with the corresponding labels of major tissue types. As seen in the figure, the human brain consists of three main tissue types, gray matter (GM), white matter (WM), and cerebral spinal fluid (CSF).[1] The WM consists of axons, tracts that transmit information between the nerves in the body and the neurons on the GM. The sheet of GM surrounding the WM is called the cerebral cortex, which is characterized by its highly convoluted surfaces. The convolution or folding of the cortex creates gyri and sulci[2] patterns as shown in Fig. 1.3, and allows the fitting of a large surface area into the restricted cranial space bounded by the skull. Anatomically, the thin cortical sheet has six cytoarchitectonic layers, and has a thickness that varies between 1–5

---

[1]Although CSF is not truly a tissue type, it is always considered as a constituent of the brain.

[2]"Gyri" is the plural of "gyrus", and refer to the ridges of the cortical fold; "sulci" is the plural of "sulcus", and refer to the valleys.

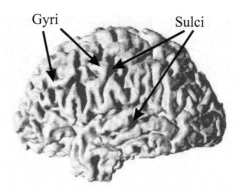

Figure 1.3: A computed cortical surface.

mm, with an overall average of approximately 2.5 mm [6–9]. In this work, we aim at reconstructing three surfaces to model the cerebral cortex — the inner GM/WM interface, the outer GM/CSF interface (also known as the pial surface), and a surface lying at the geometric center of the cortical sheet, which approximately corresponds to the cytoarchitectonic layer four. Fig. 1.4 illustrates the location of the three cortical surfaces on a 2D cartoon drawing of the brain.

1.2.2 Significance of brain cortical surface reconstruction

Segmentation of an MRI brain image into its constituent tissue types and reconstructing the cortical surfaces are important for various neuroscience and medical applications. Application areas include:

1. Visualization. Segmentation of the cortex and finding its boundary surfaces allows the use of fast and simple surface rendering techniques to fully visualize the cortical geometry. Various functional or other experimental data can also be easily overlaid on the surface display for illustration and visual analysis [10,11]. We would like to refer the reader to the website prepared by Paul Thompson[3]

---

[3]http://www.loni.ucla.edu/~thompson/MEDIA/AD/PressRelease.html

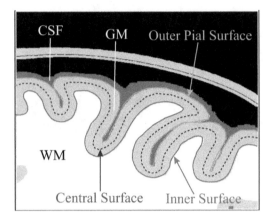

Figure 1.4: A cartoon drawing illustrating the definition of the three cortical surfaces.

for a striking example of visualizing the effect of Alzheimer's disease on cortical geometry.

2. Surgical Planning. Segmented brain images, together with a registered visualization, allow surgeons to see the 3D arrangement of anatomical structures, which helps the surgeon to plan the surgical path [12]. For example, many sulci can be used as natural pathways to gain access to pathologic structures deep inside the brain [13].

3. Surface-based Atlas. Although 3D volumetric atlases such as the Talairach atlas [14] have been widely used due to their simplicity, it has been realized that a surface-based atlas would provide a better substrate for displaying and analyzing anatomical and functional data of the brain cortex [11, 15–17]. A major advantage of a surface-based atlas for the brain cortex is that such a representation respects the intrinsic topology of the cerebral cortex as a 2D sheet, and permits a *geodesic distance* measurement between locations on the cortical surface. The Euclidean distance measure assumed in a 3D volumetric atlas can substantially underestimate the true distance along the cortical sheet, and lead to errors and misunderstanding about the localization and relationship

of structural and functional sites of the brain. In order to establish such a surface-based brain atlas, a correct and accurate cortical surface reconstruction is needed.

4. Functional brain mapping. Combining functional data (e.g. PET, fMRI, or MEG) with segmented brain anatomy helps the identification and localization of various functional areas of the brain [10]. As in the surface-based brain atlas, a reconstructed cortical surface better represents the intrinsic structure of the brain cortex, which facilitates the correct depiction of intra-cortical relationship of different activation sites as opposed to the simple Euclidean distance. The geometric information provided by a surface representation can also benefit many EEG and MEG reconstruction methods by significantly reducing the solution space [10, 18].

5. Multi-modal Registration. A reconstructed cortical surface can provide important anatomical landmarks for various 3D registration algorithms [19–24]. A direct benefit is that more accurate and anatomically meaningful registrations can be achieved.

6. Cortical Unfolding. Cortical unfolding refers to the removal of the buried folds of the cortex, revealing the entire structure of the cortex on a flat, convex, or radial surface [15–17, 25–29]. Such reconfiguration is desired for better visualization of the buried cortex and for the establishment of a standard cortical coordinate system that facilitates comparison of various functional studies across subjects. All cortical unfolding methods cited above require a topologically correct surface reconstruction of the cortex.

7. Evaluation and diagnosis of brain abnormalities. There is increasing evidence that geometric anomalies in the cortex are often associated with neurological and psychiatric disorders. For example, the loss of GM volume and enlargement of cortical sulci has been noticed in Alzheimer's disease [30]. Certain other than normal sulcal and gyral patterns in the left temporal lobe are believed to be correlated with schizophrenia [31]. In addition, it has been shown that

cortical pathologies often manifest themselves in abnormal variations of cortical thickness [32].

1.3 Difficulties of Medical Image Segmentation

There is a large body of literature on medical image segmentation, and a brief review will be provided in Chapter 2. Overall, medical image segmentation is a difficult problem, especially for the segmentation and surface reconstruction of MR brain images. In this section, we discuss several problems faced by medical image processing, in general, and MRI brain image segmentation in particular. These problems include image noise, image intensity inhomogeneity or non-uniformity, and the partial volume averaging effect.

Noise in MR images stems from several sources: thermal noise from the RF coil, dielectric or inductive losses in the patient, and noise introduced by the electronic circuitry of the imaging hardware [5,33]. For imaging applications at field strengths greater than 0.5 Tesla (which is the case for typical brain imaging), the dominant noise source is the Johnson thermal noise from inductive currents in the patient [5,33]. This noise can be well approximated as Gaussian-distributed, white, and additive [5,33]. The presence of noise causes random variations in the measured signal intensity, and limits the quality of MR images.

Image intensity inhomogeneity, also known as the *shading artifact*, refers to a smooth intensity variation of a same tissue type across the image, which is introduced by the image acquisition device. This artifact is typical in MR images and depends on several factors, which include the shape and electromagnetic properties of the subject being scanned, the spatial inhomogeneity of the magnetic excitation field, the spatial sensitivity of the radio-frequency (RF) receiver coil, and gradient-driven eddy currents. Intensity inhomogeneity causes a particular tissue to appear brighter in one part of the image and darker in another. Although this slowly-varying intensity change has little impact on human interpretation of the image, it can pose large problems for automated image segmentation methods, especially those that rely on absolute image intensity values. Fig. 1.5 demonstrates this artifact. The image slice

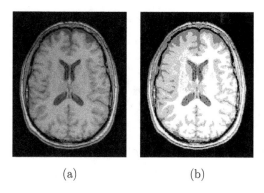

(a)   (b)

Figure 1.5: Illustration of image intensity inhomogeneity. (a) Original image with shading artifact; (b) Segmentation result using K-mean clustering algorithm.

in Fig. 1.5(a) is corrupted by a non-uniform intensity gain field, and appears brighter at bottom-right than at top-left. Due to this shading artifact, the standard K-means clustering algorithm based on the image intensity misclassifies most WM tissues as GM on the top-left part of the image.

The Partial Volume Effect (PVE) refers to a mixing of more than one tissue types in a single voxel. It arises due to the finite spatial resolution of the image acquisition system. PVE causes edge blurring at the interface of different tissue types, and reduces the accuracy and reliability of measurements taken on the images. The PVE has a large effect in MR imaging of the brain cortex, where the image resolution is limited by other considerations such as scanning time, motion artifacts, and image signal-to-noise ratio. Due to these practical limitations, a typical T1-weighted brain image volume has a spatial resolution of about 1 mm × 1 mm within-slice, and 1–1.5 mm in slice-thickness. As mentioned before, the brain cortex is highly convoluted and with an average thickness of 2.5 mm. Thus, it can be imagined that a very high percentage of the image voxels within the cortex region will be affected by the PVE.

The PVE makes it particularly difficult to properly identify the pial surface of the brain cortex. Due to the tightly folded configuration of the brain cortex (see Fig. 1.4), there are many places in the brain where the cortical GM on one side of a

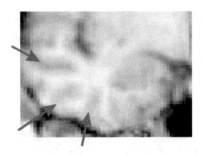

Figure 1.6: A zoomed view of a T1-weighted brain image slice. The pial matter (CSF) is invisible within the sulcal folds due to the partial volume effect. The arrows point to the PVE-blurred sulci.

sulcus (called a cortical bank) is very close to or actually touches the cortical GM on the opposite side. The PVE causes the two cortical GM banks to appear as a solid GM block, and the interface between GM and CSF becomes invisible (see Fig. 1.6). As a result, estimating the pial surface based on the image data alone would be likely to produce an over-smoothed surface without showing the sulcal folds. Such an estimate is incompatible with the anatomical knowledge that requires separate GM banks within each sulcal fold, and can cause large inaccuracies in estimating the cortical thickness and other cortical geometry measures. To resolve the PVE artifact, a cortical reconstruction method needs to take into account prior knowledge about cortical anatomy, as demonstrated in the literature [34, 35] and in Chapter 5 of this book.

1.4   Anatomical and Topological Constraints in Medical Image Segmentation

In many computer vision tasks, the image to be analyzed consists of an unknown scene with unknown objects. In contrast, in medical image analysis, the number of object components and the homology and overall geometry of each component is usually known *a priori*. Thus, a natural requirement for a successful medical image segmentation method is that it should at least be able to produce the correct object composition and topology and be consistent with the *a priori* anatomical knowledge.

As the simplest anatomical constraint, the boundary surface of a 3D anatomical object should be a valid 2D manifold[4] in other words, a simple surface. A simple surface refers to a surface without any self-intersections. Although this constraint seems trivial, not every segmentation method automatically conforms to this constraint. For example, parametric deformable models, which have been widely applied in medical image segmentation, can easily develop self-intersections (see the next section and Chapter 2 for a detailed discussion on deformable models). A recent method improves upon the traditional parametric deformable model by adding an additional constraint to avoid self-intersections [35], but the resulting method is quite time-consuming. We note that another type of deformable model, the geometric deformable model, can automatically avoid the self-intersection problem. However, existing geometric deformable models have no control of the model topology, and their segmentation results can easily violate known topological constraints.

By definition, topology refers to the invariant property of an object up to continuous deformations. For example, a circle and a triangle have the same topology. Anatomical objects typically have a known topology, and segmentation results should reflect this anatomical property. For example, many organs, such as kidney, prostate, and each hemisphere of the brain cortex, have boundary surfaces topologically equivalent to a 2D sphere. When processing the brain cortex as a whole object, its cortical surfaces are assured to have a spherical topology when the hole around the brainstem area is closed.

Generating a topologically correct cortical surface model is critical for many brain mapping applications. For example, spherical surface topology is assumed in all cortical flattening or spherical mapping approaches [15, 25, 27–29, 36]. Maintaining the correct surface topology also allows for more accurate estimation of the geodesic distance between two cortical locations, which is important for functional brain mapping [10] and building surface-based atlases [16]. In practice, topological defects such

---

[4]A 2D manifold is a topological space such that each of its points has a neighborhood that is homeomorphic to an open planar disk.

as holes or handles can easily arise due to image noise and segmentation errors. Thus, methods are desired that either can perform topology correction on an initial segmentation with the wrong topology or can guarantee the correct topology.

In addition to the simple surface and the topology constraints, there are some other anatomical constraints that must be considered for the brain cortical surface reconstruction task. For example, reconstructions for the three cortical surfaces should preserve the correct geometric relationship, and should not intersect with each other. Another constraint arises due to the partial volume effect as discussed in the previous section, that is, the segmented GM/CSF boundary should follow the folding pattern of the WM/GM boundary. All these topological and anatomical constraints are the major considerations in our design of a successful cortical surface reconstruction method.

1.5 Deformable Model based Image Segmentation

Deformable models constitute a class of popular and powerful medical image segmentation methods due to their ability to combine low-level image information with high-level prior knowledge about object shapes [37, 38]. The inherent continuity and smoothness of these models offer robustness against image noise, boundary gaps, and spurious edges in the image, and provides the potential for subpixel accuracy in delineating object boundaries. A major focus of the work presented in this book is on the modification of existing deformable model methods to improve their performance.

By definition, deformable models are elastic contours[5] defined within an image domain that can deform under the influence of internal shape forces and external image forces. The shape forces control the regularity and smoothness of the modeling contour or its closeness to a prior shape estimate, while the image forces drive the contour towards object boundaries or other desired features within an image. The contour is considered to reach an equilibrium state or to have converged when the internal forces balance out the image forces.

---

[5]In this book, we use the word *contour* to refer to either a curve or surface, and the words curve and surface are used explicitly only when the dimensionality must be clear.

Deformable models are broadly classified as either *parametric deformable models* (PDMs) (cf. [39–43]) or *geometric deformable models* (GDMs) (cf. [44–54]) according to their representation and implementation. In particular, parametric deformable models are represented *explicitly* as parameterized contours (i.e., curves or surfaces) in a Lagrangian framework. The initial deformable model introduced by Kass et al. [39] falls into the category of PDMs. GDMs, or implicit deformable models, on the other hand, are represented *implicitly* as level sets of higher-dimensional, scalar level set functions and evolve in an Eulerian fashion [55]. Geometric deformable models were introduced more recently by Caselles et al. [44] and by Malladi et al. [45].

There are pros and cons for both types of deformable models, largely depending on particular application requirements. PDMs maintain an explicit discrete sampling or parameterization of the contour, and can maintain the initial contour topology. However, frequent contour resampling is necessary during the contour deformation process in order to accurately represent the contour geometry while reducing unnecessary computational cost. Resampling can be tedious, especially in 3D. A second shortcoming of PDMs is that discrete nodal (polygonal) representation makes computation of geometric properties of the contour, such as the normal vector and the contour curvature(s), inaccurate. A third drawback of PDMs in medical image segmentation applications is that the contour can develop self-intersections, especially when segmenting structures such as the brain cortex with its highly convoluted boundary surfaces. Self-intersection violates the anatomical consistency requirement, and also renders the deformable model unstable. Some recent work addresses the self-intersection problem by adding a collision detection mechanism into the PDM framework [35]. Unfortunately, the computational demands related to self-intersection detection are very high, especially for surfaces [35]. As a result, most PDMs still neglect this step, relying instead on smooth external forces and extremely small step sizes. We note that although PDMs are typically favored in cortical surface reconstruction applications due to their ability to preserve model topology, topology correctness is truly meaningful only when self-intersection can be prevented.

Although developed much later than PDMs, GDMs have quickly gained enormous popularity due to several important advantages they offer over parametric models.

First, they are completely intrinsic and therefore are independent of the parameterization of the evolving contour. In fact, the model is generally not parameterized until evolution of the level set function is complete. Thus, there is no need to add or remove nodes from an initial parameterization or adjust the spacing of the nodes, as in parametric models. Second, the intrinsic geometric properties of the contour such as the unit normal vector and the curvature can be easily computed from the level set function. Third, GDMs prevent self-intersections inherently because of their level set representation as well as the entropy conditions imposed during level set evolution [55, 56]. Criticism about GDMs often includes the increased computational cost associated with the extra dimensionality of the embedding level set function. However, many efficient algorithms developed such as the Fast Marching Method and the Narrow Band Method [55] have largely overcome this disadvantage.

The other drawback of GDMs for our application is the lack of topology control. In GDMs, the embedded contour can freely change topology by merging or splitting or forming cavities or handles in 3D. This topological flexibility has long been claimed as a major advantage of GDMs over PDMs, and it is so desirable in some applications that methods to adaptively change the contour topology have also been developed for PDMs [57, 58]. But topological flexibility is not always desired, especially in medical image segmentation applications. As explained before, anatomical objects typically have a known topology and composition, and producing the correct topology is a major requirement rather than merely a desirable feature. Another obvious drawback of the lack of topology control is that it can easily lead to over-segmentation, resulting in the need for an additional stage of post-processing.

Clearly, it is desirable to have a deformable model that combines the advantages of both frameworks. In particular, for medical image segmentations, the deformable model should be able to produce a result with the correct topology and without self-intersections. This requirement is the primary motivation for our development of topology-preserving geometric deformable models, presented later in this book.

1.6 Major Contributions

The work presented in this book comprises the following major contributions:

1. **Multiscale, graph-based topology correction algorithm:** A method was developed for the topology correction of binary digital volumes and isosurfaces of gray-scale or floating-point valued images. The method is intrinsically 3D, and applies techniques from mathematical morphology, digital topology, and graph theory. It uses a multiscale approach and combines both foreground and background processing to optimize the detection and removal of topological defects (handles) from the original volume or surface. This method is used to produce a topologically correct result from an initial image segmentation having the wrong topology. This provides a topologically correct initialization for image segmentation based on deformable surfaces, and is a key component of the cortical surface reconstruction method presented later in this book.

2. **A topology-preserving geometric deformable model:** A family of new geometric deformable models were developed that have the ability to maintain the prescribed model topology, while retaining the other advantages of traditional geometric deformable models such as computational stability and the property of automatically avoiding self-intersections. These properties make the new deformable models very useful tools in medical image applications where topologically correct and anatomically feasible boundary segmentations are desired. This deformable model comprises another key component of our cortical surface reconstruction method.

3. **Brain cortex reconstruction method:** We present a systematic approach for the automatic reconstruction of the human brain cortex from MR brain images. Although the basic principle follows a previous method developed in our group [2], the new method makes use of the newly developed topology correction algorithm and the new geometric deformable model, and aims at obtaining a complete cortical characterization by reconstructing all three representative

surface layers of the cortex. Some additional new components were also proposed to improve the automation of the method, as well as its accuracy and robustness against the partial volume effect.

4. **Moving grid geometric deformable model:** To resolve a resolution problem related to geometric deformable models, we investigated adaptive grid techniques and developed a class of moving grid geometric deformable models. The resulting method improves the accuracy of both traditional and the topology-preserving geometric deformable models while maintaining a low computational cost. It also has the property of achieving simultaneous surface simplification and thus provides a good framework for the development of better surface reconstruction methods in medical imaging applications.

1.7 Previous Publications

Portions of this book have been previously published in peer-reviewed international journals and conference proceedings. The topology correction algorithm was published in [59, 60]. The topology-preserving geometric deformable model was published in [61–63]. Reports on the cortical surface reconstruction method and its components were published in [64–66]. Finally, a 2D version of the moving grid geometric deformable model was published in [67].

1.8 Book Organization

The book is organized as follows. In Chapter 2, we briefly review medical image segmentation techniques, provide the necessary background knowledge about deformable models, in particular the geometric deformable models, and also the background information concerning digital topology and isosurface algorithms. In Chapter 3, we present our method for performing topology correction of binary image volumes and for producing topologically correct isosurfaces from any given gray scale or floating-point valued 3D images. In Chapter 4, we present a new class of topology-preserving geometric deformable models and demonstrate its advantage over traditional deformable models in applications where a topological constraint is necessary. In Chapter 5, we present a systematic method for the automatic reconstruction of three surface representations of the cerebral cortex from MR brain images. In Chapter 6, we discuss the adaptation of a moving grid method to the geometric deformable model framework, and develop a class of moving grid geometric deformable models. Finally, we conclude in Chapter 7 with a summary of the major results of this book and a discussion of directions for future research.

18

19

Chapter 2

Preliminaries

In this chapter, we introduce the background knowledge required to understand the methods described in the next few chapters. We begin with a brief overview of existing medical image segmentation techniques, and then review the basic principles of deformable model methods. A detailed introduction to the theory and implementation of geometric deformable models is also presented. Finally, we review the basic concepts and technologies from the field of digital topology and introduce the design of isosurface algorithms.

2.1 Medical Image Segmentation Techniques

Medical image segmentation is the process of isolating relevant anatomical objects in a given medical image data set. It is an important step in almost all the applications that use medical image data: 3D visualization, surgical planning, disease diagnosis, drug evaluation, etc. An exhaustive survey of the available medical image segmentation techniques is beyond the scope of this book. There are already several good surveys in the literature [38, 68–71]. Here, we briefly summarize the major approaches that have been taken, with emphasis on deformable model based segmentation methods.

There are many possible ways to categorize the large family of segmentation methods. In the following, we broadly group them into low-level data-driven methods and high-level model-based methods. The low-level methods include thresholding, edge detection, region growing, and various clustering methods. The high-level methods include template matching, deformable models, and atlas-guided approaches. We note that quite often multiple techniques are used in conjunction with one another to fulfill a particular segmentation task. For example, a low-level clustering or edge detection approach is often used at the initialization stage of a high-level deformable model based segmentation method.

2.1.1 Low-level methods

Intensity thresholding may be the simplest segmentation method. In this approach, the image voxels are separated into object and background classes based on a chosen threshold value. The advantage of this approach is that it provides an easy and fast method of classifying image data. It is usually hard to choose the optimal threshold value however. Thus, the thresholding method is often applied interactively, such that the threshold value is adjusted "on the fly" based on an operator's visual assessment of the corresponding segmentation result. Variants of the thresholding technique include the use of spatially varying or multiple (two-stage) thresholds [72,73] and the incorporation of spatial connectivity information [74]. In general, thresholding methods are sensitive to image noise and the intensity inhomogeneity artifact.

Edge detection methods apply a gradient operator to detect abrupt changes in image intensity. The most popular gradient operators include the Marr-Hildreth, Sobel, Prewitt, and Canny operators [75]. High gradient points are considered as candidates for object boundaries, and are linked appropriately to produce the final coherent boundary representation. Edge linking methods range from the simple contour following or border tracing method [76] to more complicated dynamic programming techniques [77, 78]. Edge detection methods suffer from spurious edges, strong variations in gradient magnitudes, and gaps in boundaries. As a result, edge based methods are not guaranteed to produce a well-behaved object boundary. For example, the boundary found for an anatomical object may not even be a closed contour.

Region growing methods rely on homogeneity criteria defined in regions of the image domain, which can be derived from image intensity, texture, color, or image gradients. Starting from a given set of seed points, a region growing procedure grows each region by adding compatible neighboring points until the homogeneity criterion no longer holds. To avoid the need to place seeds, split-and-merge algorithms can be used. These algorithms start from non-uniform regions, and then subdivide or regroup them until uniform regions are obtained [79]. Image noise can affect the results and cause holes in the extracted regions, and the partial volume effect may result in separate regions being wrongly merged.

Clustering methods assign labels to image data points based on their positions in some well-chosen feature space, which can also be viewed as identifying *clusters* in the feature space. The feature space could be the one-dimensional intensity space; vector-valued features are also possible, perhaps formed by combining the intensity feature with various texture measures. Multi-channel or multi-spectral images of the same scene automatically produce a vector feature space. As a typical example, MR imaging is multi-spectral in nature due to the many contrast characteristics it can generate, e.g., T1-weighted, T2-weighted, and proton-density-weighted scans of the same subject.

Clustering methods can be further classified as either supervised or unsupervised depending on whether training data are needed or not. Unsupervised methods are usually preferred since it can be hard to get enough training data for supervised methods. Supervised methods include the Minimum Distance classifier [68], the k-Nearest-Neighbor (kNN) classifier [80], the Bayes classifier [81, 82], the Decision Tree classifier [83], and Artificial Neural Networks (ANNs) [84]. Unsupervised methods include the K-means algorithm [85], the fuzzy c-means algorithm [86], and the expectation-maximization (EM) algorithm [87]. The fuzzy c-means, the EM algorithms, and their variants have been proven very useful for the segmentation of MR brain images [88–91] because of their capability to model the partial volume effect and to simultaneously estimate the intensity inhomogeneity. Unfortunately, clustering methods do not directly produce a consistent and compact segmentation of anatomical structures; thus, further processing is required to obtain a coherent and consistent representation of object shapes. For example, the class membership or posterior probability estimates are often used as inputs to a high-level deformable model method, so that low-level data information and prior knowledge can be efficiently combined to achieve a good final segmentation [2, 92].

2.1.2   High-level methods

Although low level methods can be successful in processing high contrast, noise -free images, problems often arise when medical images are corrupted with noise and the anatomical structures to be segmented do not have clearly defined boundaries. Overcoming such difficulties often requires the incorporation of prior anatomical knowledge or object shape models in order to achieve reliable and useful segmentation results.

One way to incorporate shape knowledge is to use explicit geometric models. Although simple rigid 2D or 3D models can work well for segmenting regular, man-made objects as in machine vision applications, the flexible and variable nature of anatomical objects in medical imagery usually requires deformable templates or deformable models. In this book, we reserve the term *deformable model* to refer to the well-known 2D or 3D active contour models, which Jain et al. [93, 94] refer to as *free-form deformable models*. Such deformable models apply very generic local shape constraints such as continuity and smoothness, and thus can represent any arbitrary shape. Other more structured deformable models will be referred to explicitly as deformable template models, deformable shape models, or deformable atlas models. The methods in this second group of deformable models apply some form of global shape constraints, where the admissible shapes are strongly constrained by either prior shape knowledge, an atlas image, or the selected training samples. As a result, they are less generally applicable than active contour models.

The basic concept of active contour models was introduced in the previous chapter. The mathematical background will be discussed in more detail in the next section. In the remaining part of this section, we only discuss three globally constrained deformable models, i.e., the deformable template, the deformable shape, and the deformable atlas models.

Deformable template methods restrict the class of admissible shapes to a family described by a few parameters or by some prototype templates. For example, the parameterized template family includes the Fourier shape descriptor proposed by Staib et al. [95, 96], the deformable superquadrics by Terzopoulos and Metaxas [97] and Vemuri et al. [98], the adaptive B-splines by Figueiredo et al. [99], and the modal analysis method by Nastar and Ayache [100]. Prototype-based deformable template model was first introduced by Grenander et al. [101] in the framework of *general pattern theory*, the application of which in medical image analysis gave rise to the fascinating field of *computational anatomy* [102–104]. Other examples of the prototype template models include the bitmap boundary model by Jain et al. [93], the manually drawn outline contour model by Mignotte et al. [105], and the deformable medial primitives by Pizer et al. [106]. Like active contour models, deformable template models often interact with the image to be segmented through an energy minimization process, which balances the fit of the template to important image features with the deviation of the deformed template from the expected shape. The deviation is measured either by a probability distribution of shape parameters or by a suitable energy measure of the deformation field.

The next class of methods, known as deformable shape models or active shape models, focuses on the active learning of prior shape distributions from a set of training samples. After the example shapes are properly aligned, principal component analysis is used to generate an average shape and a set of principal modes of variation. The learned shape probability distribution is then used to constrain the admissible shape when a new image containing the expected shape is to be segmented. Active shape models were proposed by Cootes et al. [41, 107], and have become important techniques in medical image segmentation [54, 108–110]. One drawback of these methods is that it is usually hard to get a sufficient set of training samples for 3D images with complicated anatomical structures such as the brain cortex. More recent work in this area has been focused on automating the landmark generation process in building the shape models [111–113].

Deformable atlas methods warp a pre-segmented atlas image to the target image that requires segmentation. The atlas warping, or image registration, can be achieved using either linear [114] or nonlinear transformations [102, 115, 116]. If the warp is done correctly, then the target image will be segmented automatically; all structural information presented in the atlas can be transferred onto the target. Such methods make it possible to do one very detailed segmentation on one image, e.g., manually, and then apply the results to many other images. Deformable atlases provide a common reference system for studying the morphometric changes across individual subjects. However, the actual anatomical variabilities make it difficult to accurately recover the local details of the target structures with a fixed atlas image. In addition, an optimal warping may be hard to achieve, because image registration by itself is a difficult and unsolved problem that is still undergoing very active investigation.

2.2   Deformable Contour Models

As introduced briefly in the first chapter, deformable contour models, or active contour models, are object-delineating contours (curves or surfaces) that deform within a 2D or 3D image under the influence of both internal and external forces and user defined constraints. They implement a generic model-based image segmentation tool and have found applications in a wide variety of medical image segmentation tasks. Comprehensive surveys can be found in [37, 38, 117]; in this section, we introduce only the basic principles.

Mathematically, a deformable contour can be represented as a parameterized contour $C(\mathbf{p})$, with parameter $\mathbf{p} \in \Omega$, where $\Omega = [0,1]$ in 2D and $\Omega = [0,1]^2$ in 3D. For each value of $\mathbf{p}$, $C(\mathbf{p})$ is a point in 2D or 3D space, that is, $C(\mathbf{p}) = (x(\mathbf{p}), y(\mathbf{p}))$ in 2D and $C(\mathbf{p}) = (x(\mathbf{p}), y(\mathbf{p}), z(\mathbf{p}))$ in 3D. In the original formulation [39], the deformable contour is specified to minimize the following energy functional:

$$E_C = \int_\Omega E_{\text{intern}}(C(\mathbf{p}))d\mathbf{p} + \int_\Omega E_{\text{image}}(C(\mathbf{p}))d\mathbf{p} + \int_\Omega E_{\text{constraint}}(C(\mathbf{p}))d\mathbf{p},$$

where E_{intern}, E_{image}, and $E_{\text{constrain}}$ denote the internal shape energy, image derived energy, and the energy corresponding to user-supplied constraints, respectively.

E_{intern} controls the regularity (continuity and smoothness) of the contour. For example, in 2D, E_{intern} usually has the following form:

$$E_{\text{intern}} = w_1(\mathbf{p})|C_{\mathbf{p}}(\mathbf{p})|^2 + w_2(\mathbf{p})|C_{\mathbf{pp}}(\mathbf{p})|^2,$$

where $C_{\mathbf{p}}$ and $C_{\mathbf{pp}}$ denote the first- and second-order derivative of $C(\mathbf{p})$ with respect to $\mathbf{p}$, respectively. The first-order term makes the contour act like an elastic band, and is called the *tension* energy; the second-order term makes it to resist bending, and is called the *rigidity* or *stiffness* energy. Adjusting the weights $w_1(\mathbf{p})$ and $w_2(\mathbf{p})$ controls the relative importance of the tension and rigidity energy. The same concept applies to a 3D active surface model, but the formula is more complicated (cf. [118]).

The image energy term E_{image} is used to attract the contour towards desired image features. For example, in object boundary detection, E_{image} can be defined as

$$E_{\text{image}}(C(\mathbf{p})) = -|\nabla I(C(\mathbf{p}))|^2,$$

where $\nabla I(C(\mathbf{p}))$ denotes the image gradient at a contour point $C(\mathbf{p})$. There are many other possible definitions; we will explore several in this book.

The constraint energy term $E_{\text{constraint}}$ can be used to implement user interactive control in order to guide the contour towards or away from particular image locations. For example, a spring-like attraction effect can be created between a contour point $C(\mathbf{p}_0)$ and a user-defined image location $\mathbf{x}_0 = (x_0, y_0, z_0)$ by choosing:

$$E_{\text{constraint}} \propto |C(\mathbf{p}_0) - \mathbf{x}_0|^2.$$

Other forms of constraint energy also exist [39]. In this book, we aim at developing fully automatic image segmentation methods; hence, this term is never used in our applications.

Computing the Euler-Lagrange equation of the energy functional E_C produces a necessary condition that the contour C must satisfy in order to minimize the energy. That is,

$$\frac{\partial E_C}{\partial C} = 0, \tag{2.1}$$

where $\frac{\partial E_C}{\partial C}$ denotes the first-order variation [119] (a generalized gradient) of the energy functional with respect to C. Very often, energy minimization is achieved computationally through an iterative gradient-descent-like algorithm. More specifically, instead of directly solving (2.1) for the optimal contour $C(\mathbf{p})$, one can embed $C(\mathbf{p})$ into a family of contours $C(\mathbf{p}, t)$ with an additional time parameter t. One can then iteratively solve

$$
\begin{cases}
\dfrac{\partial C(\mathbf{p}, t)}{\partial t} & = \quad -\dfrac{\partial E_C}{\partial C}, \\[2ex]
C(\mathbf{p}, t = 0) & = \quad C(\mathbf{p}, 0),
\end{cases}
\tag{2.2}
$$

starting with an initial contour $C(\mathbf{p}, 0)$ until convergence. $C(\mathbf{p}, 0)$ is referred to as the *initialization* of the deformable model. Since a gradient-descent algorithm only performs a local energy minimization, the active contour model will converge to the correct solution only if its initialization is sufficiently close to the desired optimum.

The negative gradient of the energy functional in (2.2) is usually called the force or speed term of the contour deformation (people use "force" and "speed" interchangeably in the literature), and can be denoted as F_{intern}, F_{image}, and $F_{\text{constraint}}$ respectively corresponding to each of the energy terms. For example in 2D, we have

$$
F_{\text{intern}}(C(\mathbf{p}, t)) = -\frac{\partial E_{\text{intern}}}{\partial C} = -\frac{\partial}{\partial \mathbf{p}}\left(w_1(\mathbf{p})\frac{\partial C(\mathbf{p}, t)}{\partial \mathbf{p}}\right) + \frac{\partial^2}{\partial \mathbf{p}^2}\left(w_2(\mathbf{p})\frac{\partial^2 C(\mathbf{p}, t)}{\partial \mathbf{p}^2}\right).
$$

Then, the dynamic evolution equation of the contour can be rewritten as:

$$
\frac{\partial C(\mathbf{p}, t)}{\partial t} = F_{\text{intern}}(C(\mathbf{p}, t)) + F_{\text{image}}(C(\mathbf{p}, t)) + F_{\text{constraint}}(C(\mathbf{p}, t)).
\tag{2.3}
$$

Very often, different deformable models are designed by defining the force terms directly instead of starting from the energy formulation. This design strategy offers more flexibility [118], but may produce models that have no variational principle as their basis.

For the numerical implementation of the deformable model method, many methods first discretize the continuous contour into a connected set of discrete contour nodes, $C(\mathbf{p}_0, t), C(\mathbf{p}_1, t), \ldots, C(\mathbf{p}_N, t)$. The deformation equation, (2.3), is then solved at these discrete contour points; the continuous contour can only be obtained by an interpolation method such as the spline interpolation used in [39]. This discretization scheme corresponds to the class of *parametric deformable models* (PDMs), as was mentioned in Chapter 1. As also mentioned previously, such a contour discretization or sampling requires frequent adjustment of the spacing and the number of contour nodes (called reparameterization) during the deformation process, in order to faithfully represent the contour geometry and reduce numerical approximation errors. Methods for reparameterization in 2D are usually straightforward and require moderate computational overhead. Reparameterization in 3D, however, requires complicated and computationally expensive procedures. Self-intersection is another major problem of PDMs in medical image segmentation applications, which can cause instability in the numerical implementation and result in invalid object boundary representations.

The need to eliminate the requirement for reparameterization and the desire to improve the accuracy and stability of the numerical implementation of contour deformation led to the development of *geometric deformable models* (GDMs), which are the topic of the next section.

2.3   Geometric Deformable Models

Geometric deformable models (GDMs) are deformable models that are implemented using level set numerical methods [55]. In this section, we briefly review the main theory and major results of geometric deformable models.

2.3.1   Front evolution and level set theory

As can be seen in the previous section, the implementation of deformable contour models is reduced to solving the contour deformation equation, (2.3), which describes a family of evolving contours $C(\mathbf{p}, t)$, where t parameterizes the family and $\mathbf{p}$ parameterizes the given contour. This contour deformation process is in direct analogy to the front propagation problem in the computational physics literature [55,56]. In [56], Osher and Sethian proposed an Eulerian approach to study front propagation problems, which gave the now famous *level set method*. This numerical method is a highly accurate and stable method for solving front propagation problems, and its application to the solution of deformable models created the class of *geometric* deformable models [44, 45].

The basic result from front evolution theory is that the geometric shape of the contour is determined solely by the normal component of its evolution velocity, while the tangential component affects only the contour parameterization. Hence, after a possible reparameterization, the evolution equation can be written as

$$\begin{cases} \dfrac{\partial C(\mathbf{p},t)}{\partial t} &= F(C(\mathbf{p},t))\vec{N}(C(\mathbf{p},t)), \\ C(\mathbf{p},0) &= C_0(\mathbf{p}), \end{cases} \tag{2.4}$$

where $F(C(\mathbf{p},t))$ is now a generic speed function and $\vec{N}(C(\mathbf{p},t))$ is the unit normal vector (conventionally chosen to be the inward normal) along the contour $C(\mathbf{p},t)$.

The level set technique developed by Osher and Sethian [56] represents the contour $C(\mathbf{p},t)$ implicitly as the zero level set of a smooth, Lipschitz-continuous scalar function $\Phi(\mathbf{x},t)$, also known as the *level set function*, where $\mathbf{x} \in \mathcal{R}^2$ in 2D or $\mathbf{x} \in \mathcal{R}^3$ in 3D. The implicit contour at any time t is given by $C(\cdot,t) = \{\,\mathbf{x} \mid \Phi(\mathbf{x},t) = 0\,\}$. Although there are infinitely many choices of the level set function, in practice the signed distance function is preferred for its stability in numerical computations. The fast marching method proposed in [120, 121] provides an efficient algorithm for constructing the signed distance function from a given initial contour. We also follow this convention in our implementation of both the standard geometric deformable models and the new variants we develop in this book. As a simple illustration, the signed distance function of a simple closed contour shown in Fig. 2.1(a) is computed using the fast marching method and displayed as a gray-scale image in Fig. 2.1(b). The zero level set of the signed distance function gives back the original contour, as shown by the yellow curve in Fig. 2.1(b).

By differentiating $\Phi(\mathbf{x},t) = 0$ with respect to t and substituting (2.4), the following associated equation of motion for the level set function $\Phi(\mathbf{x},t)$ can be derived:

$$\begin{cases} \dfrac{\partial \Phi(\mathbf{x},t)}{\partial t} = F(\mathbf{x},t)|\nabla \Phi(\mathbf{x},t)|, \\ \Phi(C_0(\mathbf{p}),0) = 0, \end{cases} \tag{2.5}$$

where ∇ is the gradient operator and $|\nabla\Phi|$ denotes the norm of the gradient of Φ. Note that the function $F(\mathbf{x},t)$ is only defined at the contour location originally, and

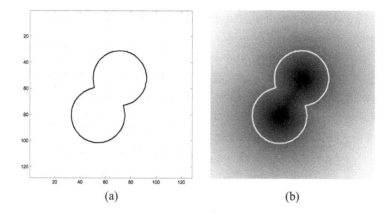

(a)   (b)

Figure 2.1: A simple closed contour (a) and its signed distance function (b). The yellow curve in (b) indicates the zero level set of the signed distance function.

hence needs to be extended to the whole computational domain (cf. [55]) in order that (2.5) applies to the whole space.

2.3.2 Geometric deformable models

Caselles et al. [44] and Malladi et al. [45] applied the above theory to the problem of image segmentation by choosing a particular speed function

$$F(\mathbf{x}, t) = g(|\nabla I(\mathbf{x})|)(c + \kappa(\mathbf{x}, t)),$$

where $g(|\nabla I(\mathbf{x})|)$, called the "stopping" term, is a monotonically decreasing function of the gradient magnitude of the image I (or its smoothed version). c is a constant inflation or deflation (depending on its sign) speed term that aims to keep the contour moving in the proper direction, and $\kappa(\mathbf{x}, t)$ is the (mean) curvature of the level set of $\Phi(\cdot, t)$ that passes through the point $\mathbf{x}$, which can be easily computed from the spatial derivatives of $\Phi(\cdot, t)$ (cf. [55]). In this way, they arrived at the following evolution equation

$$\frac{\partial \Phi(\mathbf{x}, t)}{\partial t} = g(|\nabla I(\mathbf{x})|)(c + \kappa(\mathbf{x}, t))|\nabla \Phi(\mathbf{x}, t)|. \tag{2.6}$$

We note that the above formulation was originally derived for planar curves, but it also applies to surfaces as well.

The model in (2.6) does not arise from the minimization of an energy functional as in the classical active contour models. To address this, Caselles et al. [46, 47] and Kichenassamy et al. [48, 49] derived another geometric deformable model, called the *geodesic active contour model*. The basic idea is to consider the object boundary detection as a problem of geodesic computation in a Riemannian space, according to a metric $g(\mathbf{x})$ induced by the given image I. This idea can be formally written as

$$\min_C J(C) = \min_C \int g(C(\mathbf{p}))dC, \qquad (2.7)$$

where dC denotes the arc-length in 2D or the infinitesimal area element in 3D, and $g(\mathbf{x})$ is usually chosen to be the same as the stopping term $g(|\nabla I(\mathbf{x})|)$ used in the previous model.

Minimizing $J(C)$ using a steepest descent algorithm starting from an initial contour C_0 gives the following contour evolution equation

$$\begin{cases} \dfrac{\partial C(\mathbf{p},t)}{\partial t} = (g(C(\mathbf{p},t))\kappa(C(\mathbf{p},t)) - \nabla g(C(\mathbf{p},t)) \cdot \vec{N}(C(\mathbf{p},t)))\vec{N}(C(\mathbf{p},t)), \\ C(\mathbf{p},0) = C_0(\mathbf{p}). \end{cases} \qquad (2.8)$$

This geodesic active contour model can be cast within the level set framework, yielding the level set function evolution equation

$$\begin{aligned} \frac{\partial \Phi(\mathbf{x},t)}{\partial t} &= g(\mathbf{x})|\nabla\Phi(\mathbf{x},t)|\nabla \cdot \left(\frac{\nabla\Phi(\mathbf{x},t)}{|\nabla\Phi(\mathbf{x},t)|} \right) + \nabla g(\mathbf{x}) \cdot \nabla\Phi(\mathbf{x},t) \\ &= g(\mathbf{x})\kappa(\mathbf{x},t)|\nabla\Phi(\mathbf{x},t)| + \nabla g(\mathbf{x}) \cdot \nabla\Phi(\mathbf{x},t), \end{aligned} \qquad (2.9)$$

where $\nabla\cdot$ denotes the divergence of its argument, and $\kappa(\mathbf{x},t)$ is the (mean) curvature as in (2.6).

There are many other extensions of the basic geometric deformable model in the literature (e.g., [51–54, 118, 122, 123]), which were designed either to improve the overall performance of the original model or to adapt to particular applications. Here, we consider a very general framework summarized by the following evolution equation [55, 118]:

$$\frac{\partial \Phi(\mathbf{x},t)}{\partial t} = F_{\text{prop}}(\mathbf{x},t)|\nabla\Phi(\mathbf{x},t)| + F_{\text{curv}}(\mathbf{x},t)|\nabla\Phi(\mathbf{x},t)| + \vec{F}_{\text{adv}}(\mathbf{x},t) \cdot \nabla\Phi(\mathbf{x},t), \quad (2.10)$$

where $F_{\text{prop}}(\mathbf{x}, t)|\nabla\Phi(\mathbf{x}, t)|$ is an expansion or contraction force; $F_{\text{curv}}(\mathbf{x}, t)|\nabla\Phi(\mathbf{x}, t)|$ is the part of the force that depends on the intrinsic geometry, especially the (mean) curvature $\kappa(\mathbf{x}, t)$; and $\vec{F}_{\text{adv}}(\mathbf{x}, t) \cdot \nabla\Phi(\mathbf{x}, t)$ is an advection force that passively transports the contour.

The right-hand side of (2.10) can arise from the gradient descent minimization of an energy functional, as in the geodesic active contour model of (2.9), where $F_{\text{prop}}(\mathbf{x}, t) = 0$, $F_{\text{curv}}(\mathbf{x}, t) = \kappa(\mathbf{x}, t)g(\mathbf{x})$, and $\vec{F}_{\text{adv}}(\mathbf{x}, t) = \nabla g(\mathbf{x})$. In general, however, one can choose a different form for each force term for a given purpose. As an example, we can choose $F_{\text{prop}}(\mathbf{x}, t) = R(\mathbf{x})$ to be a region force[6] (cf. [53, 118]) or a binary flow force [52], $F_{\text{curv}}(\mathbf{x}, t)$ to be proportional to the (mean) curvature $\kappa(\mathbf{x}, t)$, and $\vec{F}_{\text{adv}}(\mathbf{x}, t) = \vec{v}(\mathbf{x})$ to be a gradient vector flow force [42]. With these choices the evolution equation becomes

$$\frac{\partial\Phi(\mathbf{x}, t)}{\partial t} = \omega_R R(\mathbf{x})|\nabla\Phi(\mathbf{x}, t)| + \omega_\kappa \kappa(\mathbf{x}, t)|\nabla\Phi(\mathbf{x}, t)| + \omega_{\vec{v}}\vec{v}(\mathbf{x}) \cdot \nabla\Phi(\mathbf{x}, t), \quad (2.11)$$

where ω_R, ω_κ, and $\omega_{\vec{v}}$ are weights for the respective forces. As a simple demonstration, the model in (2.11) was applied to find the ventricle boundaries in a 2D brain image, as shown in Fig. 2.2. We omit the details for this simple 2D example. More important applications of (2.11) can be found in Chapter 5 for cortical surface reconstructions from 3D brain volumes.

2.3.3 Numerical implementation

One advantage of the geometric deformable model is that, even though the implicit contour itself can develop singularities (like cusps and corners) and can merge or split to change topology, the level set function Φ remains well-defined. Thus, one can discretize the level set evolution equation on a fixed Cartesian grid and use a finite difference scheme to robustly solve the evolution equation numerically. In order to capture the singularities that might develop along the implicit contour, Osher and Sethian [56] proposed an upwind scheme that incorporates piecewise continuous approximations to Φ and utilizes one-sided (or upwind) derivatives in the approximation

---

[6]Also known as a signed pressure force.

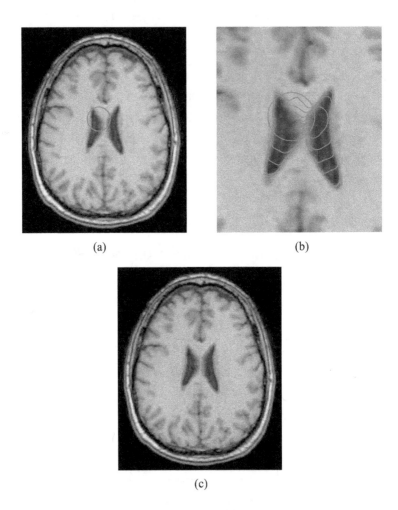

(a)

(b)

(c)

Figure 2.2: Segmentation of ventricles in a 2D brain image. (a) The brain image with the initial contour overlaid (the red circle). (b) A magnified view of the region around the ventricles, together with several plots of the evolving contour at different time steps. (c) The final boundary segmentation of the ventricles.

of $\nabla\Phi$. The scheme is numerically stable and produces an entropy-satisfying viscosity solution to (2.10).

Denote a grid point by $\mathbf{x}_i$ and the discrete time scale by t_m, where i, m are integers. The resulting level set update equation can be written as

$$\Phi(\mathbf{x}_i, t_{m+1}) = \Phi(\mathbf{x}_i, t_m) + \Delta t \Delta \Phi(\mathbf{x}_i, t_m), \qquad (2.12)$$

where $\Delta t = t_{m+1} - t_m$ is the timestep size. For the time being, we use $\Delta\Phi$ to denote the upwind finite difference approximation to the right hand side of (2.10) (see [55] for an explicit formula). Given an initial level set function $\Phi(\cdot, t_0)$, (2.12) can be used to update the level set function at successive time instants $t_{m+1}, m = 0, 1, \ldots$, until convergence. Although not explicitly computed until the end, the zero level set of $\Phi(\cdot, t_m)$, $m = 1, 2, \ldots$ represents the evolving contour(s).

As mentioned before, the forces are really only meaningful at the moving contour itself, i.e., the zero level set of Φ. Yet the update equation (2.12) applies to all values of Φ, not just those around zero. In fact, it is clear from (2.9) that in this implementation of the geodesic deformable model the forces have been "naturally" extended to apply to all level sets, not just the zero level set. By "naturally", it is meant that the same expression is used to evaluate the forces over the whole computational domain. One implication of this particular force extension is that all level sets are attracted to the desired image feature, which tends to crowd the level sets closer together ("bunching") as the iterations proceed. Because of this, periodic reinitialization of the level set function (using the fast marching method, for example) is required in order that it closely approximates a signed distance function; this improves numerical stability and accuracy of the overall computation. An alternate extension method that preserves Φ at any time as a signed distance function was presented in [55, 124], but this requires more computation per iteration and is generally much slower than this simple periodic reinitialization scheme.

There are several ways to increase the computational speed of geometric deformable models including time-implicit numerical schemes and the narrow band method. In time-implicit numerical schemes [125, 126], the level set function at the current time step is updated from its previous values by solving a system of linear equations, which means that the level set function at the grid points are updated all at once. Time-implicit schemes, however, are not compatible with the topology-preserving mechanism that we describe in Chapter 4, since they do not permit points to be controlled individually. In Chapter 4, we require a time-explicit step in order to be able to maintain explicit control of topology at each iteration. The narrow band method [127, 128] is perfectly compatible with our requirement, and in fact provides a considerable computational advantage since only a small set of grid points near the zero level set are modified during each iteration. Furthermore, the method described in Chapter 4 can be expressed as a small, but critically important modification to the standard narrow band method. For this reason, we now give the explicit steps of the narrow band implementation of a geometric deformable model.

Algorithm 2.1: Narrow Band Algorithm

1. *Initialize* — Set $m = 0$ and $t_0 = 0$. Initialize $\Phi(\cdot, 0)$ to be the signed distance function of the initial contour.

2. *Build the Narrow Band* — Find the narrow band points. These are the grid points $\mathbf{x}_i$ whose distance $|\Phi(\mathbf{x}_i, t_m)|$ is less than the user-specified narrow band width (a positive number).

3. *Update* — Set $t_{m+1} = t_m + \Delta t$. For every narrow band point $\mathbf{x}_i$, update its level set function value $\Phi(\mathbf{x}_i, t_{m+1})$ using (2.12).

4. *Reinitialize* — If necessary, reinitialize $\Phi(\cdot, t_{m+1})$ to be the signed distance function of its own zero level set.

5. *Convergence Test* — Check whether the iterations have converged. If yes, stop; otherwise set $m = m + 1$. If reinitialization was performed in Step 4, then go to Step 2 to rebuild the narrow band; otherwise, go to Step 3.

It is worth making a few comments about the narrow band method. First, we note that in Step 3, the narrow band points can be processed in an arbitrary order since each point is updated using function values from the previous time-step. Second, reinitialization of the level set function is periodically required not only to prevent "bunching" as described above, but also to prevent the zero level set from moving out of the current narrow band (cf. [55]). Third, the topology of the embedded contour is normally free to change in an arbitrary fashion during the evolution of Φ. This means that the topology of the final contour is ordinarily unpredictable; images with clutter or noise can very easily produce unexpected topological results involving multiple objects, nested objects, or handles (which are found only on surfaces). This lack of topology control makes the standard geometric deformable model unsuitable for many medical image applications where topology correctness is a major concern. As described before, a major contribution made in this book is to develop a new class of topology-preserving geometric deformable models, which will be presented in Chapter 4.

2.4 Digital Topology

Digital topology is the study of the topological properties of digital images. Its results provide a sound mathematical basis for image processing operations such as image thinning, boundary following, and region growing. In this book, the concepts and principles from the digital topology field serve as an important basis for the topology correction method and the topology preserving geometric deformable model that will be presented in the next two chapters. Thus, in this section, we present a brief review of the relevant concepts and principles. A more complete and rigorous introduction can be found in [129]. We note that although some generalizations of digital topology exist that deal with gray-scale images [130], in this book we always refer to binary-valued digital images when discussing issues related to digital topology. Such binary-valued images are typically obtained by thresholding a gray scale or floating-point valued image.

Traditionally, the domain of a digital image S is a set of rectangular array points. Without loss of generality, the array points can be assumed to be indexed by integer valued coordinates. As a result, the image domain can be considered as a subset of $\mathcal{Z}^2$ in 2D, or of $\mathcal{Z}^3$ in 3D, where $\mathcal{Z}$ stands for the set of integers.

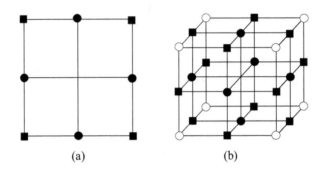

Figure 2.3: (a): 2D neighborhoods; (b) 3D neighborhoods.

The study of digital topology begins with the concepts of neighborhood and adjacency. Two neighborhood definitions are commonly used in 2D, the 4-neighborhood and the 8-neighborhood; and three types of neighborhoods are defined in 3D: the 6-neighborhood, the 18-neighborhood, and the 26-neighborhood. Their definition can be described by two distance measures. Let $\mathbf{x}$ and $\mathbf{y}$ denote generic image points, with coordinates (x_1, x_2) and (y_1, y_2) respectively if in 2D, and coordinates (x_1, x_2, x_3) and (y_1, y_2, y_3) respectively if in 3D. The two distance measures are defined as:

$$D_1(\mathbf{x}, \mathbf{y}) = \sum_{i=1}^{M} |y_i - x_i|,$$

and

$$D_\infty(\mathbf{x}, \mathbf{y}) = \max_{i=1,\ldots,M} |y_i - x_i|,$$

where $M = 2$ in 2D and $M = 3$ for the 3D case. We further define the following neighborhoods:

$$V_1^k(\mathbf{x}) = \{\, \mathbf{y} \mid D_1(\mathbf{x}, \mathbf{y}) \leq k \,\},$$

and

$$V_\infty^k(\mathbf{x}) = \{\, \mathbf{y} \mid D_\infty(\mathbf{x}, \mathbf{y}) \leq k \,\}.$$

Then in 2D, the 4-neighborhood of a point $\mathbf{x}$ is $N_4(\mathbf{x}) = V_1^1(\mathbf{x})$, and the 8-neighborhood is $N_8(\mathbf{x}) = V_\infty^1(\mathbf{x})$. In 3D, the 6-neighborhood of a point $\mathbf{x}$ is $N_6(\mathbf{x}) =$

$V_1^1(\mathbf{x})$, the 26-neighborhood is $N_{26}(\mathbf{x}) = V_\infty^1(\mathbf{x})$, and the 18-neighborhood is $N_{18}(\mathbf{x}) = V_1^2(\mathbf{x}) \cap V_\infty^1(\mathbf{x})$. The above neighborhood definition includes the point $\mathbf{x}$ itself. The neighborhood without the central point is denoted by $N_n^*(\mathbf{x}) = N_n(\mathbf{x})\backslash\{\mathbf{x}\}$, where $n = 4$ or 8 in 2D, and $n = 6, 18$, or 26 in 3D. Two points $\mathbf{x}$ and $\mathbf{y}$ are said to be n-adjacent or n-connected with n as above if $\mathbf{y} \in N_n^*(\mathbf{x})$; $\mathbf{y}$ is also called an n-neighbor of $\mathbf{x}$. The 2D neighborhoods are illustrated in Fig. 2.3(a), where the four dark circles are the 4-neighbors of the central point, and all four dark circles and four dark squares constitute the 8-neighbors of the central point. The 3D case is illustrated in Fig. 2.3(b), where the filled circles denote the 6-neighbors of the central point. The 18-neighbors include the 6-neighbors plus the points denoted by the dark squares. The 26-neighbors include all the 26 points surrounding the central point, which includes the open circles.

An n-path is a sequence of points $\mathbf{x}_0, \mathbf{x}_1, \ldots, \mathbf{x}_k$ such that $\mathbf{x}_i$ is n-adjacent to $\mathbf{x}_{i-1}$ for $1 \le i \le k$. If each point of a n-path is n-adjacent to only its successor (if any) and its predecessor (if any), then the n-path is called a simple path. If $\mathbf{x}_0 = \mathbf{x}_k$, then the path is called closed.

A point set $X \subset S$, where S denotes a binary image, is n-connected if an n-path in X can be found between every pair of points of X. Given an arbitrary point set $X \subset S$, an n-connected component of X is a set $Y \subset X$ which is n-connected and no point in Y is n-adjacent to any other point of X, i.e., Y is maximal. We denote the set of all n-connected components of X by $\mathcal{C}_n(X)$, and the set of all n-connected components of X that are n-adjacent to a point $\mathbf{x}$ by $\mathcal{C}_n(\mathbf{x}, X)$.

In order to avoid a connectivity paradox, different connectivities, n and $\bar{n}$, must be used in a binary image comprising an object (foreground) X and a background $\bar{X}$. For example, in 2D, if n is chosen to be 4, then $\bar{n}$ must be 8, and vice versa. In 3D, (6,18), (18, 6), (6, 26) and (26, 6) are four pairs of compatible connectivities.

The topology of a set $X \subset S$ can be characterized by its Euler number $\chi(X)$. We first consider a 3D image S. In this case, $\chi(X)$ equals to the number of connected components of X plus the number of its cavities minus the number of its handles. The notion of a cavity is easy to define; it is a connected component of $\bar{X} = S\backslash X$ that is surrounded by X. For example, assume X denotes the foreground of the digital image S that does not have any boundary points of S (we can always enlarge the domain of S to satisfy this assumption). Then the cavities of X are the connected background components that are not connected to the image boundary. The notion of a handle is not simple to define, but the presence of a handle in X can be detected whenever there is a closed path in X that cannot be deformed in X to a single point without breaking the path.

In the 2D case, the above notions for cavities and handles are conflicting. For convenience, in 2D it is usually assumed that there are no cavities, and an isolated background connected component inside a foreground region is considered to be a handle of the foreground region. This convention makes the above formula for the Euler number $\chi(X)$ still applicable. That is, $\chi(X)$ equals to the number of connected components minus the number of handles in 2D. Note that, clearly the topology of X depends on the digital connectivity rule specified on X. Furthermore, a digital object X and its complement $\bar{X} = S \backslash X$ will have exactly the same number of handles under a pair of compatible connectivities n and $\bar{n}$.

We now introduce an important concept from the digital topology: the *simple point*. The notion of a simple point is essential for all image transformations that must preserve topological features, a typical example of which is the image thinning or the image skeletonization algorithms. We will see that it is also an essential part of the topology preserving deformable model we propose later in this book.

By definition, a point in a binary image S is called a *simple point* if changing the value at this point does not change the topology of the image S; that is, adding the point to the foreground or removing it to the background does not change the number of connected components, the number of cavities, or the number of handles in both the foreground and the background.

A nice property of the simple point concept is that whether a point is a simple point or not can be fully determined from the configuration of its immediate neighborhood (8-neighborhood for 2D and 26-neighborhood for 3D). Several different algorithms for simple point determination have been proposed in the literature [129, 131, 132]; the most efficient approach is the one proposed by Bertrand et al. [131, 132]. This method relies on the definition of a geodesic neighborhood and a topological number.

The original definitions appear in separate papers for the 2D case and the 3D case (cf. [131, 132]). Here, we summarize them into the following two definitions.

Definition 1 (Geodesic Neighborhood) *Let $X \subset S$ and $\mathbf{x} \in S$. The geodesic neighborhood of $\mathbf{x}$ with respect to X of order k is the set $N_n^k(\mathbf{x}, X)$ defined recursively by: $N_n^1(\mathbf{x}, X) = N_n^*(\mathbf{x}) \cap X$ and $N_n^k(\mathbf{x}, X) = \cup\{N_n(\mathbf{y}) \cap N_M^*(\mathbf{x}) \cap X, \; \mathbf{y} \in N_n^{k-1}(\mathbf{x}, X)\}$, where $M = 8$ in 2D and $M = 26$ in 3D.* ∎

Definition 2 (Topological Numbers) *Let $X \subset S$ and $\mathbf{x} \in S$. The topological numbers of the point $\mathbf{x}$ relative to the set X are: $T_4(\mathbf{x}, X) = \#\mathcal{C}_4(N_4^2(\mathbf{x}, X)$ and $T_8(\mathbf{x}, X) = \#\mathcal{C}_8(N_8^1(\mathbf{x}, X)$ in 2D; and $T_6(\mathbf{x}, X) = \#\mathcal{C}_6(N_6^2(\mathbf{x}, X))$, $T_{6+}(\mathbf{x}, X) = \#\mathcal{C}_6(N_6^3(\mathbf{x}, X))$, $T_{18}(\mathbf{x}, X) = \#\mathcal{C}_{18}(N_{18}^2(\mathbf{x}, X))$, and $T_{26}(\mathbf{x}, X) = \#\mathcal{C}_{26}(N_{26}^1(\mathbf{x}, X))$ in 3D, where $\#$ denotes the cardinality of a set.* ∎

Intuitively, a n-connected neighbor of point $\mathbf{x}$ belongs to its geodesic neighborhood $N_n^k(\mathbf{x}, X)$ if there is a path in X of length no greater than k between the neighbor and the given point. The topological numbers are the numbers of connected components within certain geodesic neighborhoods. We note that in the above definition of topological numbers in the 3D case, there are two notations for 6-connectivity. This follows the convention introduced in [131], wherein the notation "6+" implies 6-connectivity whose dual connectivity is 18, while the notation "6" implies 6-connectivity whose dual connectivity is 26. This new notation is just for convenience as it permits a compatible digital connectivity pair to be uniquely specified given only one connectivity rule (the foreground connectivity, for example). It should be clear from the above definitions that the topological number for 6-connectivity must be computed differently depending on whether the associated connectivity rule is 18 or 26.

Topological numbers are useful for classifying the topology type of a grid point. For example, they are used to define interior points, isolated points, border points, curve points, surface points, etc. in a digital object [133]. We will also use the topological numbers to define a new *nice point* criterion in our topology correction algorithm.

The topological numbers make it easy to characterize a simple point. It is proven in [131] that a point $\mathbf{x}$ is *simple* if and only if $T_n(\mathbf{x}, X) = 1$ and $T_{\bar{n}}(\mathbf{x}, \bar{X}) = 1$, where $(n, \bar{n})$ is a pair of compatible connectivities. The condition is easy to understand. For example, suppose $\mathbf{x} \in X$ and $T_n(\mathbf{x}, X) = 0$, then the deletion of $\mathbf{x}$ will remove an

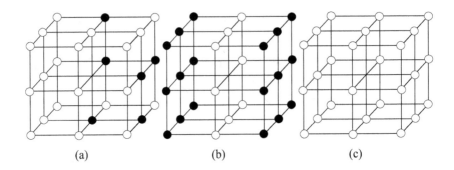

Figure 2.4: Simple and non-simple point examples. $n = 6$ for black points and $\bar{n} = 26$ for white. (a): a simple point, $T_n = T_{\bar{n}} = 1$; (b) a non-simple point, $T_n = 2$, $T_{\bar{n}} = 1$; (c) a non-simple point, $T_n = 0$, $T_{\bar{n}} = 1$.

n-component of X. Suppose $\mathbf{x} \in \bar{X}$ and $T_n(\mathbf{x}, X) = 2$, then adding $\mathbf{x}$ to X will either reduce the number of n-components of X by one, or create a handle in X. Thus, $\mathbf{x}$ is a simple point if and only if there are exactly one connected foreground component and one connected background component in the neighborhood of $\mathbf{x}$. The reason for using the geodesic neighborhoods is explained in [131, 132]. Some examples of simple and non-simple points together with the topological numbers for each case are shown in Fig. 2.4, where the central point is the point under consideration.

A straightforward computation of the topological numbers requires counting the number of connected components within the specific geodesic neighborhoods, which is the approach we take in our current implementation. A more efficient approach is to build a look-up table beforehand to store the topological numbers for each possible configuration, which, however, can take up a large memory for the 3D case since the table would have 2^{26} entries. Another approach proposed by Robert and Malandain [134] is based on the what-so-called *binary decision diagrams*. It is very efficient and avoids the use of large look-up tables, but its implementation is quite complicated.

2.5 Isosurface Algorithm

Isosurface algorithms also play an important role in medical imaging applications. For example, isosurfaces are very effective in illustrating the spatial relationship between different structures. They can also be combined with low level image segmentation methods to create surface models of various anatomical objects. Our interest in isosurface algorithms arises due to the need to extract the implicit contour from the embedding level set functions, and to compute isosurfaces from an initial fuzzy segmentation of brain images. Although the design of isosurface algorithms is a well studied problem, it still takes some care to correctly implement a working isosurface algorithm without producing undesirable artifacts. In our application, it is also important to make sure that the computed isosurface correctly reflects the topology of the underlying volume. Thus, in this section, we present the necessary background about the isosurface algorithms and their implementation. We focus on the popular *marching cubes* (MC) algorithm [135]. Later in Chapter 3, we propose a variant of the MC algorithm that is consistent with the digital connectivity rules specified on a binary volume.

Formally, an isosurface is defined as a surface that connects all the points of a 3D space that have the same function value associated; this function value is called the *isovalue*. Methods used to extract the isosurface from a trivariate function or a discrete 3D volume data set are called the *isosurface generation algorithms*, which are also known as *implicit surface tilers* in the computer graphics literature.

We first note that the most common surface representation for describing a generic surface is with connected polygons, triangles being the simplest form. Modern graphics hardware can render such polygonal surfaces very efficiently and, hence, most isosurface extraction techniques have concentrated on this representation. Note also that polygonal or triangular meshes are also the typical surface mesh format used in parametric deformable models.

Among various isosurface algorithms, the MC algorithm is the most simple and the most popular one as well. It was first presented in 1987 by Lorensen and Cline [135] as an efficient method to create polygonal (usually triangular) surface representations from a scalar field sampled on a rectilinear grid. The algorithm works by first partitioning the data space into cubical (or rectilinear) cells, with the cell vertices being the grid points. It then processes each cube one at a time, and approximates patches of the isosurface within each cube by polygon pieces. After all the cubes are processed, the polygon patches are naturally joined together to form the final isosurface representation. Such a polygonal surface can be easily turned into a triangular mesh by converting each polygon into one or more triangles.

With this scheme, the isosurface construction is reduced to surface tiling within each individual cube. For this purpose, the algorithm first assigns a binary label to each vertex of a cube, based on the relative polarity of the data value at the vertex as compared against the given isovalue. For example, a "1" is assigned to the vertex if its data value is greater than or equal to the isovalue; otherwise, a "0" is assigned. Then a cube is said to intersect with the isosurface if not all of its vertices have the same label or polarity. The surface intersection is computed at each edge of the cube that joins two vertices with opposite labels, usually by a linear interpolation of the original vertex values. Intersections within each cube face are connected to form face contours (line segments), which are combined sequentially with face contours from other faces to form (possibly nonplanar) polygonal patches that approximate the isosurface within the cube.

Before we proceed further, we want to point out that the MC algorithm makes two assumptions or simplifications regarding the behavior of the isosurface within each cube, although the true surface can, in general, have arbitrary complexity. First, the isosurface cannot have isolated components that are fully contained inside a cubical cell. Second, there is exactly one surface intersection at a cube edge that connects oppositely labeled cell vertices, and there is no intersection if an edge connects two vertices of the same polarity. These assumptions are reasonable for high data sampling resolution; in other words, the data variation should be small with respect to the cell size.

Under the above assumptions, the surface tiling of a cube is quite simple. Since each cube vertex has one of two possible labels, there are only $2^8 = 256$ ways an isosurface can intersect a cube. The corresponding surface patch generation can be

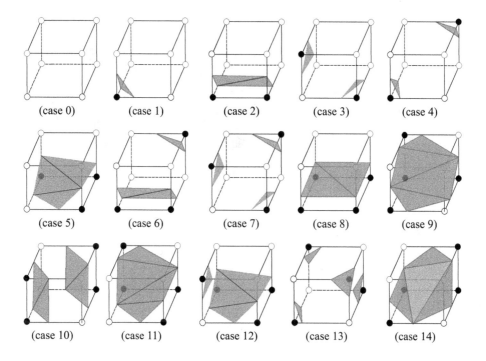

Figure 2.5: The 15 major cases of the MC algorithm.

built into a lookup table with 256 entries. Such a table only stores the topology of the polygonalization for each case. The actual coordinates of the surface-cube intersections are computed dynamically by linear interpolation using the actual data values. In the original MC paper [135], the 256 cases are further reduced into 15 *major* cases by complementary and rotational symmetry. They are illustrated in Fig. 2.5.

One problem found in the early implementation of the MC algorithm is related to the topology of the surface, and is often referred to as the topology inconsistency problem. The problem happens when neighboring cubes make inconsistent connectivity decisions at their common face, as shown in Fig. 2.6(a). This inconsistency problem causes holes in an otherwise closed surface as shown in Fig. 2.6(b), which is the result from a free, publicly available isosurface software. The correct surface tessellation is

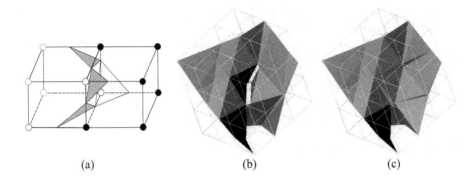

(a)   (b)   (c)

Figure 2.6: (a) Inconsistent tiling across neighboring cubes. (b) Hole in the surface. (c) Correct surface tessellation.

shown in Fig. 2.6(c), a result that was generated using our own implementation of the MC algorithm. The problem is actually due to an inherent ambiguity in the surface tessellation within a cube. In other words, the way in which an isosurface intersects a cube is not always unique. Two types of ambiguities exist in the MC algorithm: one or more faces of a cube is ambiguous, or the entire body of the cube is ambiguous. These ambiguities are illustrated in Fig. 2.7.

The above topology inconsistency problem can be addressed by making sure that an ambiguous face is tessellated in the same way in the two cubes that share the face. But even this solution is not unique. Various methods have been proposed to deal with this problem, and a survey can be found in [136]. For example, some methods apply rules that imply certain preferred polarity, e.g., always separate the two vertices with "0" labels, or the other way around. Other methods decompose each cube further into a set of tetrahedra, and apply the so-called *Marching Tetrahedra* (MT) algorithms. At first glance, it appears that the MT algorithm has no ambiguity in the tiling of each tetrahedron; however, the original ambiguity is actually transferred to the ambiguity in the tetrahedra decomposition. A different decomposition will result in a different surface topology. We did not pursue the MT approaches due to two major problems. First, it is difficult to apply the traditional digital topology concepts on the decomposed grid. Second, the decomposition introduces additional edges. As a result,

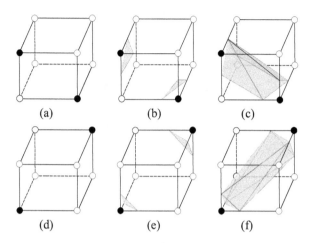

(a)   (b)   (c)

(d)   (e)   (f)

Figure 2.7: Ambiguity in isosurface tiling. (a) An ambiguous face; (b) and (c) are two possible tilings. (d) An ambiguous cube; (e) and (f) are two possible tilings.

MT algorithms usually produce huge surface meshes, and thus a mesh simplification procedure is usually required as a postprocessing stage, which by itself is a difficult problem.

Another method to remove the ambiguity from the MC algorithm was developed by Natarajan [137]. This method actually goes a further step beyond the topology consistency problem. It actually tries to achieve a topology correctness objective, that is, to produce a surface mesh with the same topology as the true isosurface. This goal is impossible to achieve in general without additional assumptions or prior knowledge, however. In this method, it is assumed that the underlying function is locally trilinear in each cube. Thus, the method computes two types of *saddle points*, which correspond to the critical points of the underlying function. One type is called the *face saddle points* that are computed at each ambiguous face; and the other is the *body saddle points* that are computed at an ambiguous cube. The saddle points can also be labeled by comparing the (trilinearly) interpolated function value at their location against the given isovalue. After that, ambiguity removal can be accomplished by selecting the tiling that connects the vertices with the same label as

46

that of the saddle point. For example, the tiling in Fig. 2.7 (f) will be chosen if the body saddle point has the same label as the black points; and Fig. 2.7(e) otherwise. The trilinear assumption may not hold in general, however. Thus, their claim of guaranteed topology correctness must be interpreted with care.

Another problem that is often neglected in MC algorithms is the creation of singularities in the computed surface mesh. There are three types of singularities: a singular vertex, a singular edge, and a singular face (cf. Fig. 2.8). By definition, a singular edge is an edge in the polygonal or triangular mesh that is shared by more than two polygonal or triangular faces. A singular face is a polygonal or triangular face that shares more than one edges with another face. To define the singular vertex, we need the notion of the *link* of a vertex. The *link* of a vertex v is the union of all the edges that do not contain v but belong to a polygonal or triangular face that has v as one of its vertex. Then, a vertex is singular if its link is not topologically equivalent to a circle or a line segment.

The cause for the singularity problem in the MC algorithm is actually very simple: it happens when the data value at a grid point exactly equals to the chosen isovalue. In such cases, the surface intersections at adjacent cube edges will collide into the same cube vertex, and cause one or more edges or faces in the surface triangulation to be degenerated to a single point. Unfortunately, many free or commercial MC software packages do not explicitly handle this problem, and the resulting mesh often has singularities. The images in Fig. 2.8(a)–(c) were produced from one such public domain MC software package. As we can see, the existence of the singularities prevents the surface mesh from being a valid 2D manifold and makes it appear as if it has self-intersections.

There are two approaches to avoid the singularity problem in practice. The first method requires data preprocessing. Specifically, one can detect whether a data value is exactly equal to the given isovalue, and slightly adjust the data value if this happens. The surface meshes in Fig. 2.8(d)—(f) were produced by this method. Different adjustment (increasing or decreasing) of the data value, however, can result in a different surface topology. Therefore, these adjustments need to be done with caution, or by making use of additional knowledge about the surface being sought.

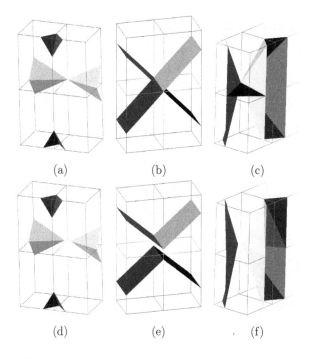

(a)   (b)   (c)

(d)   (e)   (f)

Figure 2.8: (a), (b), (c): singular point, edge, and face, respectively, from a free MC software; (d), (e), (f): the correction by our MC implementation.

The second approach to get around the singularity problem is to choose an isovalue that is known to be different from all possible data values. For example, it is better to use a floating-point non-integer isovalue when defining the isosurface of a digital gray-scale image.

The MC algorithm introduced above has an analog in 2D called the *Marching Squares* (MS) algorithm. MS can be used to extract the isocontours from a 2D image data set. The MS algorithm shares a similar principle as the MC method, but the implementation is simpler due to the reduction in dimensionality. For example, one only needs to deal with one ambiguous case, the ambiguous square, which is a square whose two diagonals have opposite polarity. The implementation can be easily deduced by direct analogy to 3D MC, thus, we will not present the details of the MS algorithm here.

2.5.1 Topology of surface meshes

As a follow-up to the isosurface algorithm, we introduce here the topological characterization of a triangulated surface mesh, e.g., the output of an MC algorithm. The topology of a connected surface mesh is fully characterized by its Euler number, denoted by χ. As the symbol signifies, the Euler number here is the same as the Euler number of a point set we discussed in the previous section. But, for a triangulated surface mesh, there exists a simple formula to compute its Euler number [138]:

$$\chi = N_V - N_E + N_F, \tag{2.13}$$

where N_V, N_E, and N_F are the numbers of vertices, edges, and faces, respectively, of the surface mesh.

From the Euler number, the so-called *genus* g of the surface mesh [138] can be computed:

$$g = 1 - \chi/2. \tag{2.14}$$

For a closed and orientable surface, g denotes the number of handles of the surface. Such a surface is topologically equivalent to a sphere when $g = 0$, which is how we check the topology correctness of the reconstructed cortical surfaces in our method. Note that neither the Euler number nor the genus provides any information about the size or location of a handle. In fact, the detection and localization of handles can be very difficult; and many complex algorithms have been recently developed to effectively detect and remove surface handles, as will be surveyed in Chapter 3.

Chapter 3

Graph-based, Multiscale Topology Correction Algorithm

Producing the correct topology is an important requirement in medical image segmentation applications. For example, in cortical reconstruction, the computed cortical surface representation must be a simple closed surface that is topologically equivalent to a sphere. A reconstructed cortical surface without the correct spherical topology is incompatible with the known cortical geometry, and can lead to incorrect interpretations of local structural relationships and prevent cortical unfolding. Unfortunately, most image segmentation methods do not guarantee the topology correctness of the final results, and topological errors such as handles or tunnels can easily arise in the segmentation process due to imaging artifacts such as noise and the partial volume effect. As illustrated in Fig. 3.1, the terms "handle" and "tunnel" actually refer to complementary views of the same topological defect: a handle is associated with a tunnel, and a tunnel is a handle in the background if the roles of the interior (foreground) and the exterior (background) of the surface are interchanged.

Currently, most existing cortical surface reconstruction algorithms either ignore the topology requirement or rely on a manual postprocessing to correct the topology of the initial segmentation results. Manual detection and correction of topological defects can be difficult and very time-consuming, especially for complicated surfaces like the brain cortex [36,139,140]. As a result, typically only large errors are corrected

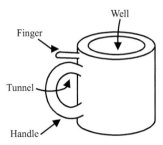

Figure 3.1: Illustration of relevant topological features.

and smaller ones are still ignored [36].

In this chapter, we describe an automatic topology correction method, which we refer to as the *graph-based topology correction algorithm* (GTCA). GTCA applies techniques from mathematical morphology, digital topology, and graph theory to detect and remove handles. It also makes use of a multiscale approach and two types of topology correction filters to achieve an optimal correction for each handle, and thus reduces the total changes necessary for topology correction. As a result, the topology corrected volume remains identical to the original except for small changes made locally to remove handles. The core method is designed to work on binary volumes, but it can be combined with a few extra steps to correct isosurfaces in graylevel volumes. This method serves as a key component in the cortical surface reconstruction method we describe in Chapter 5. Finally, we also propose a *connectivity consistent* isosurface algorithm that guarantees that the isosurface computation is consistent with the digital topology principle applied in GTCA.

The chapter is organized as follows. In Section 3.1, we review the related work in the literature, and discuss their advantages and disadvantages and relationship to our method. In Section 3.2, we present the GTCA algorithm for the topology correction of binary volumes. In Section 3.3, we introduce the connectivity consistent marching cubes isosurface algorithm. We then discuss in Section 3.4 the generation of GTCA for the topology correction of isosurfaces from general gray-scale or floating-point valued 3D images. We demonstrate the performance of the algorithm in Section 3.5. Finally, we discuss some of the considerations in a real application, and then summarize the chapter.

3.1 Related Work

Although topology correctness is an important requirement in medical image segmentation, it has drawn the attention of the research community only quite recently. Actually, several topology correction algorithms were proposed at roughly the same time as our method was first published [59]; to date, however, there have been no systematic comparison among various algorithms. We note that topology correction is a topic of general interest; therefore, we also review here techniques available in other literature, mainly in digital topology and computer graphics.

Generally, the available topology correction methods can be grouped as either volumetric methods [2, 59, 60, 140–147], i.e., methods that work on a volume data; or surface-based methods [148, 149], i.e., methods that detect and remove handles directly on an explicit surface mesh. In the following, we survey first the surface-based methods, and then the volumetric methods.

3.1.1 Surface-based topology correction methods

There are two approaches in the literature that operate directly on the explicit triangular meshes [148,149]. The method reported in [148] aims to replace the manual editing procedure used in [36] with an automatic method. The method first inflates the original surface mesh onto a sphere. Then, the existence of handles are detected as overlapping triangles on the inflated surface. The detected handles are finally removed by re-tessellating the surface mesh to remove the overlapping triangles. The success of the method largely depends on the first surface inflation step, because the same handle can result in different amount of triangle overlapping after the inflation and false overlapping may also exist due to improper implementation or insufficient inflation. The method applies a two-step iterative inflation procedure to minimize the final surface overlapping. The process by itself takes about one hour as reported by the authors. The final mesh re-tessellation step is also quite complicated, and may cause self-intersection in the final surface mesh. It is also time-consuming since it requires the building of a list of edges with one entry for every pairwise combination of vertices in a defective region. Thus, the method can be very slow for surfaces with a large number of handles, which is common in brain cortex reconstruction.

The second surface-based approach comes from the computer graphics literature [149]. The method aims to remove small handles on a surface mesh. It does this by simulating wavefront propagation within a certain neighborhood surrounding each mesh vertex. A handle that is smaller than the size of the neighborhood is detected when the wavefronts meet. It is then broken by cutting the mesh along a closed path that encloses the handle and re-tessellating the mesh to seal the resulting holes. This correction will always fill the tunnel associated with a given handle rather than cutting the handle itself (cf. Fig. 3.1), which may not be the best strategy, especially with long, thin handles. Furthermore, the method is computationally intensive, and the final correction strongly depends on the vertex used to identify the defect. Again, it is hard to ensure the manifold property of the final mesh due to the surface re-tessellation needed.

3.1.2   Volumetric topology correction methods

The majority of available topology correction methods are volumetric methods. Typically, the ultimate goal of a volumetric method is also to produce a topologically correct surface representation [2, 59, 60, 140, 143–145, 147]; thus, it is usually followed by an isosurface algorithm to get the final surface mesh. The design of the isosurface algorithm is rarely discussed, however. As we saw in the previous chapter, the common isosurface algorithms have inherent topology ambiguities and can easily ruin the volumetric topology correction results. Therefore, we believe that volumetric correction methods must consider isosurface algorithm design as well. In addition, all the volumetric methods except for the median filtering approach by Xu et al. [2] require a binary volume as input. As a result, a graylevel image volume must be first binarized before these methods can be applied. After topology correction and object boundary tessellation, further smoothing of the surface mesh is required in order to reduce the staircasing artifact of the surface that arises due to the data binarization [140, 145]. This extra surface smoothing may generate new topological errors, however. In Section 3.4, we design a new isosurface topology correction procedure that avoids the need for surface post-smoothing by making use of the original image data in the isosurface computation. The same procedure can be used with any of the volumetric topology correction methods, and thus addresses an important weakness of these methods. In the following, we survey these methods roughly in the order of their first appearance. We include the *homotopic deformable region* method proposed by Mangin et al. [13] as a possible topology correction method, since some later proposed topology correction methods are based on similar principles.

The homotopic deformable region method [13] starts with an initial region with the required topology (typically a single voxel), and then grows it by adding points that will not change the region topology. As we introduced in Chapter 2, such points can be found by the *simple point* criterion. Note that if a binary object originally has handles, then this method can be used to generate a new object without handles. The final effect is that the remaining non-simple points that are not grown back form "cuts" in the original handle locations. The problem with this simple approach is that the result, i.e., the locations of the final cuts, strongly depends on the order in which the points are grown starting from the initial region. As an extreme example, it is possible for a volume that has only one small handle to be grown in such a way that the resulting volume has a long cut at a very undesirable position. This kind of artifact is obvious in the results presented in [13], where there are unnatural cuts in the middle of the brain volume.

The method described in [141, 146] can be viewed as a dual to the homotopic deformable region method. Instead of growing simple points from inside the object, this method starts with a convex hull of the original object, and keeps removing simple points that are not part of the original object. The effect is that instead of cutting off handles, the method always fills up the tunnels (called "holes" by the authors) associated with a handle (again, cf. Fig. 3.1). In order to optimize the locations of the "blocks" that fill up the tunnels, the method orders the removal of the points in the

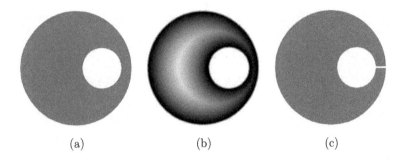

(a)   (b)   (c)

Figure 3.2: (a) A 2D ring-shaped object of nonuniform thickness. (b) The distance function computed from each object point to the object boundary (the two red circles); brighter values indicate greater distances. (c) Homotopic region growing with distance ordering breaks the ring at its thinnest part.

initial convex hull by their distance to the hull boundary. Such a distance ordering helps the final blocks be roughly centered within the object and helps reducing the size of the final blocks.

Distance ordering will not always help, however; and its effect tends to be over-rated in the literature [140]. We emphasize this point here because the distance ordering sounds very attractive, and people are often misled by it. This may be because, in 2D, the distance from the object boundary can always help in finding the thinnest part of a nonuniform, ring-shaped object. For example, the authors of [140] used a 2D illustration like that in Fig. 3.2 to demonstrate the benefit of the distance ordering. In this 2D case, a homotopic region growing algorithm that grows the object points in a decreasing order of their distance value can indeed break the ring at its thinnest part, as shown in Fig. 3.2(c). Unfortunately, this same effect does not hold in 3D. As an example, suppose that the ring-shaped object in Fig. 3.2(a) is actually a 3D object that is totally flat in the third dimension. In this case, the distance at every object point to the object boundary (a closed surface in this case) is all roughly equal to zero. As a result, ordering the points by their distance value would have no effect at all.

In [2], Xu et al. proposed an iterative median filtering approach to correct the topology of the WM isosurface. The method iteratively smoothes an initial WM segmentation until its boundary surface has the spherical topology. Unfortunately, the method is not guaranteed to converge. In fact, the median filtering can create new handles that are not in the initial volume. Another drawback is that the median filtering smoothes the entire volume, resulting in large amount of unnecessary modification. A similar method exists in the computer graphics literature [142], where morphological filters (dilation and erosion) are used to smooth the original volume. It has the same drawbacks as the median-filtering approach.

A very efficient volumetric topology correction method was developed by Shattuck and Leahy to remove all the handles from a binary WM segmentation of brain MR images [143–145]. Instead of region-growing or global filtering, their approach examines the connectivity of the binary WM volume across the 2D slices in order to find regions that give rise to incorrect topology. Then, rather than simply removing these regions, their method carefully edits the underlying volume to make the smallest possible changes (within the limits of their overall approach) that will correct the topology. Their method is elegant and effective, but there is still room for significant improvement. First, the authors acknowledge that their handle cuts are not very natural since they can only be oriented along the Cartesian axes. They also describe a particular topological problem in which "slice duplication" is required. Finally, their approach applies to only one particular digital connectivity rule, i.e., the 6-connectivity for the digital object, and has not been generalized for any other digital connectivity. This limits the performance and appearance of the final result.

The other topology correction method developed for the cortical surface reconstruction of MR brain images was proposed in [140]. Similar to the method of Mangin et al. [13] and of Aktouf et al. [141, 146], the method does not directly search for handles. Instead, it performs the same type of region growing as in [13] to find the subset of object points that form no handles. The method improves the results by adding the distance ordering to the region growing procedure. But the authors improperly used a 2D illustration to demonstrate the benefit of the distance ordering of their 3D method, as we have mentioned above. A further improvement made in this paper is to perform a second region growing in the background, which corresponds to the implementation of the hole-closing method of Aktouf et al. [141, 146]. The method then tries to find the corresponding corrections for each handle, and select the one that requires less volume modification. However, the final implementation is simplified due to the difficulty in getting the exact correspondence.

Very recently, Wood et al. [147] proposed another algorithm to remove handles in an isosurface from a volume data. The method finds the handles by incrementally constructing and analyzing a surface Reeb graph. The graph construction is very similar to that of Shattuck and Leahy method, and is performed by making axis-aligned sweep through the volume. But the graph nodes are the surface patches between two image planes and the intersecting contours of the surface with each image plane. Handles correspond again to the cycles in the graph. After handles are detected, a shortest surface loop is found for each handle. Instead of directly editing the surface to remove handle, which the authors acknowledge can result in non-manifold structure and cause mesh self-intersections, the method first converts the surface loop into the volume, and then does the modification on the volume data. A shortcoming of the method is that the handle removal procedure can introduce new handles, and thus lead to a "halting" problem. Thus, the method may be suitable only for topology simplification, i.e., removing only small sized handles.

The GTCA method we proposed [59, 60] is similar to the method by Shattuck and Leahy [143–145] in that it also detect handles by graph analysis, but our graph construction and editing procedures are quite different. In addition, our method is intrinsically three-dimensional, and "cuts" are not forced to be oriented along cardinal axes. It does not require the introduction of half-thickness slices, and any (consistent) digital connectivity definition can be used. A final distinction of our approach is that correct topology can be assured through application of either foreground or background filters alone. This procedure would result in either handles being cut or tunnels being filled exclusively, which may not be a good option in brain mapping, but may be useful for other applications.

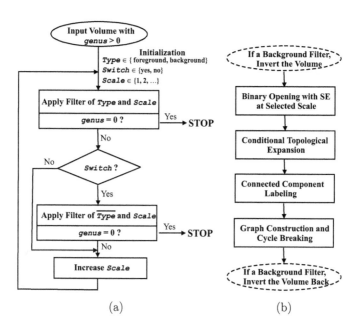

Figure 3.3: Topology correction algorithm: (a) flowchart of the algorithm, and (b) flowchart of a foreground/background filter.

3.2 Graph-based Topology Correction Algorithm

Our graph-based topology correction algorithm (GTCA) aims to remove all the handles in a binary volume. We assume that the binary volume has a single connected foreground object with no cavities.[7] A block diagram of the algorithm is shown in Fig. 3.3(a). As described above, there are two ways to correct each handle: either directly cut it or fill the associated tunnel (cf. Fig. 3.1 and Fig. 3.12). As a result, there are two classes of filters that GTCA can apply to correct the topology of an input volume: foreground filters and background filters. Handles removed by a background filter correspond to tunnels filled in the original volume. The filters are also designed with spatial scales, that is, only detecting and removing handles with a certain size.

---

[7]Cavities, unlike handles, are background regions completely surrounded by the object; they are easily removed using standard region-growing.

The meaning of the scale or the size will become clear later. Since, in general, small corrections are desirable, the two types of filters should be applied alternatively and with gradually increasing scales. That is, all "thin" handles are first cut, and all "narrow" tunnels are first filled; the filter scales can then be increased to cut or fill larger handles or tunnels. The scale is increased until all the handles or tunnels in the original volume are removed. As shown in Fig. 3.3(a), the user is also allowed to exclusively use only one type of filters, which may be desirable for certain applications. We note that since the two types of filters operate on the foreground and the background respectively of the same digital volume, a pair of compatible digital connectivity rules must be chosen for both of them, which yields an n-connectivity foreground filter and an $\bar{n}$-connectivity background filter.

Fig. 3.3(b) shows the flowchart of a foreground or background filter. The background filter is the same as the foreground filter except that it works on the complement of the original volume and assumes an $\bar{n}$-connectivity instead of the n-connectivity used in the foreground filter. As shown in Fig. 3.3(b), each filter consists of four major steps. The basic idea behind the development of each step is further illustrated in Fig. 3.4. Basically, a morphological opening operator is first applied to separate the digital object (or the inverse object if a background filter is applied) into two groups, the *body* parts and the *residue* parts. A conditional topological expansion (CTE) procedure, similar to the homotopic region-growing procedure of Mangin et al. [13], is used to replace residue parts that do not involve handles. A graph is then constructed by analyzing the connectivity between the body and the residue pieces, and handles are detected as *cycles* in the graph. A minimum set of residue pieces are then removed to break the cycles in the graph, thus removing handles in the volume.

We now describe each step in detail. We note that certain parts of the algorithms presented in this section could, in principle, be implemented in parallel. We have not considered the implications of parallel implementation, however, and therefore the algorithms should be viewed as sequential.

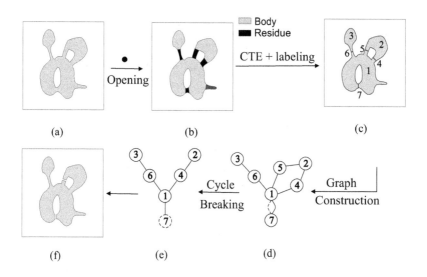

Figure 3.4: Illustration of the basic idea.

3.2.1 Binary morphological opening

We use morphological opening as a multiscale analyzer to detect handles at different scales. The morphological opening of object F with structuring element B removes all parts of F that are smaller than B, in the sense that they cannot contain any translated replica of B. We call the structuring element (SE) used at the smallest scale (scale 1) the *basic structuring element*. The structuring element at the scale k is obtained by $k - 1$ successive dilations of the basic structuring element with itself. In practice, we use a digital ball of radius one — i.e., an 18-connected neighborhood plus the center point — as the basic structuring element. This gives the ability to make very small topological corrections that are more isotropic than the slightly smaller 3D cross (another logical choice for the basic structuring element). The shape of the basic SE is not critical to the success of the algorithm although the computation time and the final result will be different. For example, a 3D cross, which has only seven points, might yield a result with fewer changes to the digital volume, but it might also take longer to compute because it would require more scales. In any case, the resulting filtered volume will have the correct topology.

As illustrated in Fig. 3.4(b), the opening operation divides the foreground object into two classes. Points that are in the resulting (opened) image are called *body* points, and points removed by the opening operator are called *residue* points. If there are regions within a handle that cannot fit the structuring element, then the handle is broken into body and residue parts. Other parts of the object, such as fingers (cf. Fig. 3.1), can also be removed or broken into different body and residue parts as well. The next step of our method seeks to transfer as many points as possible from the residue back to the body without adding a handle.

3.2.2 Conditional topological expansion

Examination of Figs. 3.4(c)–(f) leads to the idea that handles might be broken by detecting cycles in a graph comprising body and residue pieces and discarding the smallest residue piece in each cycle. Unfortunately, on a complicated shape such as a white matter segmentation, morphological opening removes far more voxels than just those required to break the handles, no matter what structuring element is used. Typically, the residue set comprises many connected components, several of which are large, complicated shapes. Also, the opening can actually *create* handles in the body component. Thus, introducing a graph-based cycle-removal procedure at this stage is likely to discard unnecessarily large pieces of the object and generate new topological problems.

Our solution is to transfer as many points as possible from the residue back to the body, without introducing handles. Specifically, we grow the body set by successive dilation, but only add those points, which we refer to as *nice points*, that come from the residue and do not adversely affect the topology. A point is *nice* if when added to the body it neither replaces nor creates a handle on the body. We refer to the entire procedure as *conditional topological expansion* (CTE). Before describing the algorithm, we first explain the criterion for defining *nice* points.

Whether a point is nice or not can be decided locally using a criterion similar to that of *simple points* in the digital topology literature (cf. [129, 131, 133, 150, 151]

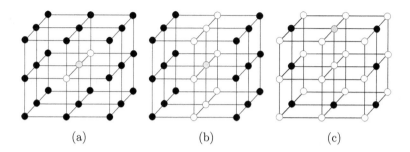

Figure 3.5: Illustration of the nice point criterion. In each figure, the gray point represents the residue point under consideration, the dark points represent body points, and the white points represent background points. In these figures, the gray point is nice in (a) and not nice in (b) and (c).

and Chapter 2). Whereas the addition of a simple point to the body is guaranteed to preserve the exact topology of the body, the addition of a nice point is allowed to fill a tunnel in the body. The use of the nice point concept is necessary because morphological opening can introduce tunnels in the body, and we want CTE to be able to fill them back up. While a simple point must preserve two topological criteria, a nice point only need preserve one criterion. Denote the set of body points by X, and let $T_n(x, X)$ be the topological number as defined in Section 2.4 of Chapter 2. From [131] (page 1010, Property 5), we have the following property:

Proposition 1 (Nice Points) *Let $x \in \bar{X}$ and suppose we add x to X. If $T_n(x, X) = 1$, then it is equivalent to say that the n-components of X are preserved and no n-handles/tunnels are created in X (and no $\bar{n}$-handles/tunnels are created in $\bar{X}$).*

Therefore, if x is a residue point that is n-adjacent to the body X, then it is *nice* if and only if $T_n(x, X) = 1$. Fig. 3.5 illustrates some examples of both nice points and non-nice points. Fig. 3.5(a) shows a case where a spurious tunnel has been created by a morphological opening. Since the gray (residue) point is originally part of the object, it should be added back to close the "false" tunnel. Note that because the gray point will change the topology when added to the body, it is clearly not a *simple* point.

By adding all the nice points back to the body, we can fill in all the false tunnels created by the opening operation. The cuts on true handles also become thinner; but they never disappear since the condition $T_n(x, X) = 1$ guarantees that adding x does not create handles in the new set $x \cup X$. Conditional topological expansion is performed using the following iterative procedure:

Algorithm 3.1 (Conditional Topological Expansion (CTE)):

  1. Find the set V of residue points that are n-adjacent to the body point set X.

  2. For each point $x \in V$, if $T_n(x, X) = 1$ then label it as a nice point.

  3. Find and label all the connected components in the set of nice points.

  4. Take the largest connected component, and relabel the points in it as new body points.

  5. If no point changed its label in Step 4, then stop; otherwise, go to Step 1.

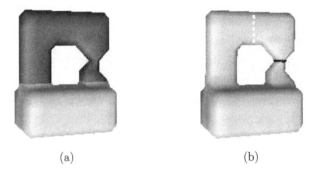

(a)   (b)

Figure 3.6: Illustration of CTE on a simple handle (surface rendering). (a) Original body (light) and residue (dark) after opening; (b) the final cut (dark) after CTE. The dashed line illustrates a non-optimal cut position.

Notice that in Steps 3 and 4 we only grow the largest connected component of nice points at each iteration instead of adding all of the nice points found in Step 2 to the body. The reason for this is to make sure that the final "cuts" — i.e., the final residue points that are not added back to the body — are positioned at the thinnest parts of the handles. This is illustrated in Fig. 3.6. In Fig 3.6(a), the darker shaded piece represents the residue after a morphological opening operation while the lighter shaded piece represents the body. The dotted line in Fig. 3.6(b) illustrates where the final cut would be if all the nice points were added back to the body after each conditional dilation. The dark line illustrates where the actual cut is placed using CTE. CTE can be made computationally efficient by using a first-in-first-out queue data structure [152] (and this is what our computer implementation does). We note that the previously mentioned distance ordering would not be able to distinguish the points along the dark line from that of the dotted white line, because the distances at these points to the background are all equal to zero (since they touch the background).

3.2.3 Connected component labeling

After CTE, any tunnels in the body that were created by morphological opening are filled in, and the remaining residue pieces form thin "cuts" that separate body components. This situation is illustrated in Figs. 3.4(b)–(c). Removing all the remaining cuts would certainly eliminate all the handles at this scale, but would also disconnect large portions of the body that we refer to as *fingers*, such as the parts labeled "6" and "3" in Fig. 3.4(c). Detecting and removing cuts that belong to handles and rejoining to the body those that are not part of handles is the aim of the graph analysis to be described in the next section. It turns out, however, that without further analysis of the remaining residue pieces, graph analysis might lead to unnecessary removal or, worse, the accidental inclusion of handles. In this section, we prepare for graph analysis by grouping the body and residue points into sets of connected components with distinct labels. We then compute the number of connections between each pair of body and residue components. When multiple connections are found, they are broken in order to break the corresponding handle(s). Special care is taken both to detect and break handles inside a residue component and to merge suitable residue components in order to avoid false cycles in the subsequent graph analysis. The overall processing strategy described in this section is illustrated in Fig. 3.7. We note that the final set of body and residue components become the nodes for the graph analysis described in the following section.

We begin by labeling the connected components of body points using n-connectivity; these form the *body connected components* or BCCs. Each residue point that

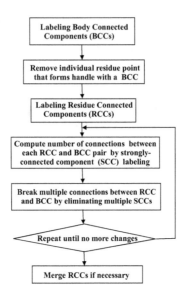

Figure 3.7: Connected component labeling and connection analysis.

forms a handle by itself with a single BCC is then removed (changed to background). These are the residue points x for which $T_n(x, X) > 1$ for some BCC X (see Fig. 3.5(c) for an example). This prevents residue connected components that are merged to the body later from forming handles that could not be detected by graph analysis. In some unusual configurations, a point removed in this step would not have actually formed a handle in the merged body. In this case, however, the last step of our algorithm (another CTE after graph analysis) adds these points back to the body.

Next, we compute the n-connected components in the remaining residue points; these form the *residue connected components* or RCCs. We must now compute the number of connections between each RCC and each of its adjacent BCCs. This computation is important because an RCC being connected to a BCC more than once indicates that there is at least one handle formed between them (e.g., see the nodes labeled "1" and "7" in Fig. 3.4(d)). The way we define the number of connections between an RCC and an adjacent BCC can be considered as a generalization of

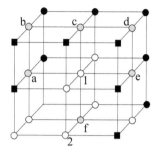

Figure 3.8: Illustration of the strong and the weak connectivity definitions (n=18). The gray points belonging to one RCC, the dark disks and the squares represent points belonging to two separate BCCs, and the rest are background points. It can be seen that a handle exists in the RCC.

the definition of topological numbers, which characterize the number of connections between a single point and its adjacent object components. This generalization leads to the concept of *strong connectivity* and *strongly connected component (SCC) labeling* as will be presented later. A subtlety exists when a handle is entirely contained within the RCC itself, as illustrated in Fig. 3.8. In this case, calculation of the number of connections between the RCC and its adjacent BCCs does not reveal the "hidden handle". The definition of a *weak connectivity* is aimed to resolve this problem. We found that if a handle is contained fully in the RCC but not in the BCC as in Fig. 3.8 (otherwise, the handle is not yet broken by the opening at the current scale), then there will be two neighboring points in the RCC that are not *weakly connected* but would be assigned to the same SCC (e.g., points with label a and f in Fig. 3.8). Thus, by removing one point from each non-weakly connected pair of neighboring points, we break handles within an RCC. We first present the two definitions (which are new as far as we know):

Definition 1 (Strong Connectivity) *Let $X, Y \subset S$ and S being a digital image. Two points $x_1, x_2 \in X$ that are n-adjacent to Y are **strongly n_k-connected** with respect to Y if $x_1 \in N_n^k(x_2, X)$ (or equivalently, $x_2 \in N_n^k(x_1, X)$) and their geodesic neighborhoods of order k inside Y intersect each other — i.e. $N_n^k(x_1, Y)$ and*

$N_n^k(x_2, Y)$ *share at least one common point.*

Definition 2 (Weak Connectivity) *Let $X, Y \subset S$. Two points $x_1, x_2 \in X$ that are n-adjacent to Y are* **weakly** n_k**-connected** *with respect to Y if there exists another point x_3 in X that is strongly n_k-connected to both x_1 and x_2.*

In the above definitions, k is chosen with respect to n as in the definition of topological numbers. For example, if n is 6^+, then k is 3. We note that strong connectivity implies weak connectivity.

An illustration of the above definitions is shown in Fig. 3.8. Suppose we consider the strong or weak connectivity relationship among the gray RCC points with respect to the BCC consisting of all the dark squares, and assume that the digital connectivity rule is $n = 18$. It is easy to check that the pairs such as (a, b), (b, c), (c, d), (d, e), and (e, f) are all strongly-connected pairs of residue points. Points a and f are 18-neighbors to each other and both 18-adjacent to the BCC, but they are not weakly-connected by the above definition. This signals a hidden handle inside the RCC itself. We can break the handle by removing either point a or f to background. Note that if the point with label 1 is also a residue point, then the handle does not exist, but then a and f become weakly-connected. Another variation is when point 2 is a foreground point, and thus belongs to the BCC of dark squares. In this case, the handle is contained in the BCC also, which says that the handle is not yet broken at the current scale. Whether we can detect the handle in the RCC is no longer a relevant issue.

Now let R_i be an RCC and B_j be a BCC that is n-adjacent to R_i. The number of connections between R_i and B_j is defined to be the number of *strongly connected components* (SCCs) formed with respect to B_j by the points in R_i that are n-adjacent to B_j. There are handles formed between R_i and B_j if R_i is connected to B_j more than once or, equivalently, if the points of R_i that are n-adjacent to B_j form more than one strongly connected components under the strong connectivity definition. Thus, after SCC labeling, if multiple SCCs exist within the RCC, we remove all but the largest one in order to break the handles formed between the RCC and the BCC under consideration. As noted above, during the SCC labeling process, we use the weak-connectivity criterion to detect hidden handles, and break them when found.

In particular, we perform the *strongly connected component labeling* (in an RCC R_i with respect to a BCC B_j) in the following way (note that we need only consider the points of R_i that are n-adjacent to B_j). We start with an unlabeled point in R_i that is adjacent to B_j and assign to it a new SCC label. Consider all its n-connected neighbors that are adjacent to B_j. Add a neighbor to the SCC if it is strongly connected. If the neighbor is not weakly connected then relabel it as background. Repeat with another neighbor of the SCC until no more neighbors can be added into it. Then, start from the beginning again to grow another SCC if possible. We remark that there is some arbitrariness in the specific result of the above algorithm as to which point to remove in a non-weakly connected pair of neighbors. Thus, the result of this algorithm is not guaranteed to be unique.

If more than one SCCs exist in R_i with respect to B_j — i.e., R_i is connected to B_j more than once — we keep only the largest SCC, removing all the others by turning them into background. After removing all but the largest SCC, each RCC is now connected to a BCC only one time at most. This step breaks the simple cycles formed by one BCC and one RCC in a connection graph like the one between BCC1 and RCC7 in Fig. 3.4(d). Since modifying an RCC with respect to one BCC may change the connection between the RCC with other BCCs, we repeat the SCC removal until no more changes are made. This procedure can also split an RCC into several disjoint parts. If this happens, we assign additional labels to each of the new residue components.

Before proceeding to graph-based handle detection, it is necessary to consider the merging of two or more RCCs. The reason for this is illustrated in Fig. 3.9(a), where $n = 6$ is assumed. In this figure, the dark points belong to the body while the gray points belong to the residue. The numbers beside the points indicate the respective BCC/RCC labels. If a graph were formed having one node per label and one edge per connection, the graph would contain the cycle 1-3-2-4-1. Graph analysis would require that either RCC 3 or 4 be removed in order to break the cycle, an apparent handle. Yet careful scrutiny of the figure shows that in reality the body and residue points taken together form a solid object without any handles. No residue need be

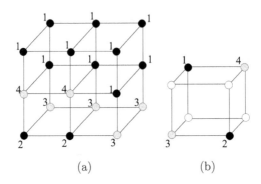

Figure 3.9: Necessity of merging RCCs. (a) 6-connectivity; (b) 18-connectivity.

removed since there is no handle to break. A similar situation can occur in the case of 18-connectivity, as illustrated in Fig. 3.9(b).

To resolve the problem, we merge the RCCs that represent the same cut between two body components. Two RCCs are said to represent the *same cut* with respect to two BCCs if the two RCCs are 18-connected at the face (if $n = 6$) or 26-connected at the cube (if $n = 18$) where the separation between the two BCCs occurs, such as RCC3 and RCC4 in Fig. 3.9(a) or 3.9(b). It is easily seen that in such cases, there can be no background path passing through the junction where the four components (two RCCs and two BCCs) meet. Thus, the two RCCs need to be merged as one single RCC since the cycle otherwise formed by the four components does not represent a true handle. In our implementation, we merge two RCCs R_i and R_j if there are two points $x \in R_i$ and $y \in R_j$ such that $x \in N_{26}(y)$ and x and y have two common n-neighbors that belong to two distinct BCCs. An RCC can be merged with more than one RCCs if it satisfies this criteria with each one of them.

3.2.4   Graph construction and cycle breaking

After considerable preparation, we are now in position to build a graph whose nodes represent the RCCs and BCCs and whose edges represent the connections between them, as illustrated in Fig. 3.4(d). Note that at this stage, there can be at

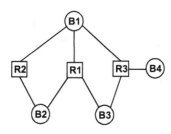

Figure 3.10: An example of a connection graph. Suppose RCC R1 is larger than R2 and R3.

most one edge between an RCC node and a BCC node. That is, cycles (handles) involving one RCC and one BCC with two or more edges between them, like BCC1 and RCC7 in Fig. 3.4(d), are already broken in the previous step by removing multiple SCCs. The remaining handles appear as cycles in the graph that are formed by more than two nodes. The graph analysis in this step aims to find such cycles and break them by removing one node from each cycle. Because of the conditional topological expansion, it is reasonable to assume that the RCCs are much smaller in size than the BCCs. Accordingly, our strategy is to remove one RCC from each cycle in order to break it, which breaks the corresponding object handle in the volume. Since we break cycles by removing *nodes* from the graph rather than *edges* as in [143,144], the maximum spanning tree algorithm (see [152]) cannot be applied in our approach. A different strategy must be used.

One strategy, which we employed in our earlier work [59], is to identify a cycle (in random order) and break it by removing the smallest RCC belonging to it. This simple approach, however, can result in unexpectedly large changes to the volume. For example, in the case illustrated in Fig. 3.10, R2 would be removed first if the cycle R1-B1-R2-B2-R1 were found first and R2 were smaller than R1. Later, R3 must be removed in order to break the cycle R3-B1-R1-B3-R3. Unfortunately, these steps cause B4 to be disconnected from the other BCCs, and this might correspond to a very large change to the volume if B4 is large. It is clear from the figure that we could have actually removed R1 to break both cycles, and no BCC would be disconnected.

70

A better strategy for breaking cycles is based on building cycle-free subgraphs. In this approach, we start by identifying RCCs that we cannot remove without disconnecting a BCC. R3 in Fig. 3.10 is such an RCC, for example, since its removal would disconnect B4. We refer to these RCCs as *leafnodes* of the graph. The key observation here is that B4 is connected to the rest only through R3. Thus, instead of removing RCCs from the original graph to break cycles, we try to build a maximum subgraph without any cycles (a maximum subtree) starting from leafnodes.

In the following algorithm, the RCCs and the BCCs are labeled separately. The label of an RCC is taken from the set {*unvisited, visited, deleted, leafnode*}. The label of a BCC is a number that indicates a subtree label.

Algorithm 3.2 (Subtree Growing Algorithm):

0. Label all the RCC nodes of the graph as **unvisited**, *set* **subtreelabel** *= 0.*

1. Find each RCC node that is the only **unvisited** *RCC node connected to a BCC node, and relabel it as a* **leafnode**.

2. If all the RCC nodes are labeled as either **visited** *or* **deleted**, *then stop. Otherwise, find the largest* **leafnode** R_i. *If there are no* **leafnodes**, *find the largest* **unvisited** *RCC node* R_i. *Relabel* R_i *as* **visited**.

3. Check the subtree labels of all the BCCs B_j, $j = 1, 2, \ldots, m$ *that are connected to* R_i. *If none of them are assigned a subtree label yet, then increment* **subtreelabel**, *and assign it to* B_j, $j = 1, 2, \ldots, m$. *If only one of them is labeled, then assign its subtree label to the other* B_j's. *The remaining possibility is that two or more of the* B_j's *are labeled and have distinct subtree labels. In this case, merge these subtrees as one, and assign (or reassign) the merged label (e.g., the smallest label) to all the* B_j's.

4. For each **unvisited** *or* **leafnode** *RCC, check whether it has two or more connected BCCs that have the same subtree label. If so, the RCC forms a handle with this subtree and is relabeled as* **deleted**.

5. Go to Step 1.

After subtree growing, the new object is reconstructed by putting together all the BCCs and RCCs except those RCCs that are labeled as **deleted**. It is easy to check that this algorithm correctly removes R1 in the graph in Fig. 3.10, and our experience is that it correctly handles the vast majority of cases. In rare occasions, however, it can happen that more than one subtrees exist after the algorithm stops. In this case, the original object is split into disjoint parts with one or more `deleted` RCCs connecting them. Ideally, one would like to connect the subtrees so that no body component is lost; but the development of a systematic approach for this process turns out to be a challenging task. It involves splitting one or more `deleted` RCC into appropriate pieces, some of which are removed to break the handles while others are kept so that the subtrees can be jointed together. We have no algorithm for doing this at present. Instead, for these cases we simply remove all the `deleted` RCCs and retain the largest resulting subtree as the reconstructed object. In our experiments, this situation occurs very infrequently and this simple strategy has never brought about a drastic change to the corrected volume. We also note that removing a whole RCC node can sometimes remove good points if the points do not belong to the edges of the cycle to be broken. We run a final pass of CTE after the graph analysis to bring these points back, which will be discussed in the next section.

3.2.5 Final stages

There are several steps that must be performed after graph reconstruction. First, it is usually possible to append points that were unnecessarily removed during the connected component labeling and the graph analysis. To do this we apply another pass of CTE using Algorithm 3.1 with the new object as the body set and the removed points as the residue set. Second, if the present filter is a background filter, the volume is inverted so that background becomes foreground and vice versa. Third, we check the topology of the resulting volume by first constructing a surface tessellation of the digital object and then computing the genus of the surface mesh (cf. Chapter 2); this approach is simpler than directly computing the Euler number of the binary volume. Note that the surface tessellation algorithm must make sure that the surface topology to be consistent with that of the underlying digital object. For this purpose, we designed a *connectivity consistent Marching Cubes* (CCMC) algorithm, which is to be presented in the next section.

If the genus of the surface tessellation is found to be zero, then the topology of the new volume is correct, and we stop GTCA. Otherwise, the proposed algorithm either switches to the opposite filter (background vs. foreground) at the same scale (if not already applied) or increases the scale of the current filter, and repeat the topology correction on the new volume (see Fig. 3.3(a)). The algorithm is guaranteed to converge because at some scale, the morphological opening must completely break all the handles, and the CTE and the graph algorithms that follows can then produce a handle-free new object.

3.3   Connectivity Consistent MC Algorithm

As discussed in the previous section, in the design of GTCA, a method is needed to check the topology of the output object, and to stop the algorithm when the topology is correct. For simplicity, we chose to perform this check by computing the genus of a surface tessellation of the object. It is thus required that the surface tessellation be topologically consistent with the underlying digital object. For example, if the object has no handles, its surface tessellation must be topologically equivalent to a sphere.

When the GTCA method was initially designed [59,60], we proposed to apply the saddle-point MC algorithm (cf. Chapter 2) to perform the surface tessellation on the binary volumes, and suggested that the surface tiling can be made to be consistent with any digital connectivity rules by properly selecting the isovalue. Basically, for 0-1 valued binary volumes where "1" indicates object, we must set the isovalue less than 0.25 to be consistent with the 26-connectivity; set it between 0.25 and 0.5 to yield 18-connectivity; and set it above 0.5 to yield 6-connectivity.

Later, in the development of the topology-preserving geometric deformable models (to be presented in the next chapter), we encountered the need to design a suitable isocontour algorithm that can faithfully recover a *digitally* embedded contour topology from the embedding level set function. In this problem, the contour is embedded as the zero level set (i.e., zero-isocontour) of a level set function, and is assumed to have the same topology as the boundary of a digital object delineated by the contour on the computational grid (hence the term "digitally embedded topology"). The research effort there led to the design of the *connectivity consistent Marching Cubes*

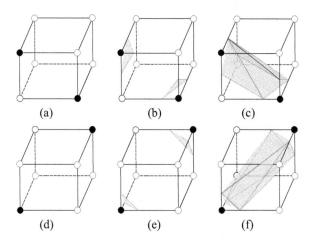

Figure 3.11: Connectivity-consistent MC algorithm. (a) An ambiguous face. (b) Tiling for 6-connectivity. (c) Tiling for 18- or 26-connectivity. (d) An ambiguous cube. (e) Tiling for 6- or 18-connectivity. (f) Tiling for 26-connectivity.

(CCMC) algorithm described in [61,63]. We later realized that the CCMC algorithm can also be used for the surface tessellation of the binary object studied in GTCA. This algorithm is actually better suited than the saddle-point MC modification since its design is directly based on digital connectivity principles and it does not limit the isovalue selection. The CCMC algorithm also makes it possible to design the isosurface topology correction algorithm to be presented in the next section. Thus, we present the CCMC algorithm here, instead of delaying it to the next chapter.

As introduced in Chapter 2, the major difference between various different MC algorithms lies in how they choose between the two possible tilings for each ambiguous case. The same conclusion applies to the design of the CCMC algorithm we propose here. For convenience, we repeat the illustration for the ambiguous face and cube cases in Fig. 3.11.

With the knowledge about the digital connectivity definitions, we can easily see that the different tilings actually correspond to different digital connectivity rules. For example, the tiling in Fig. 3.11(b) implies that the black points are 6-connected and the white points are either 18- or 26- connected. The tilting in Fig. 3.11(f) implies that the black points are 26-connected and the white points are 6-connected.

The CCMC algorithm can be described as follows: in this algorithm, the coordinates of surface intersections are still computed through linear interpolation (which gives sub-pixel resolution), but which surface tiling to choose depends on the given digital connectivity. In particular, we choose the tilings in Figs. 3.11(b) and 3.11(e) for the corresponding ambiguous cases if the black points are assumed to be 6-connected while the white points are either 18 or 26-connected. If the black points are assumed to be 26-connected, then Figs. 3.11(c) and 3.11(f) should be used instead. As can be expected, the tilings for unambiguous cases are the same as in the standard MC algorithm.

To apply the CCMC algorithm to get the surface tessellation of the digital object, any isovalue between 0 and 1 can be used. The pre-chosen digital connectivity rule for GTCA need also be supplied as an input to the CCMC algorithm. For the purpose of checking the genus of the surface mesh, the true coordinates of the surface mesh nodes need not be computed. Our CCMC implementation provides the option to omit the interpolation computation in order to save the computation time. However, to extract the final topology-corrected surface as in the isosurface topology correction algorithm of the next section, the true isovalue and the interpolation step must be applied to retain accurate surface geometry.

The corresponding connectivity consistent isocontour algorithm in 2D is named the *connectivity consistent marching squares* (CCMS) algorithm. This algorithm is not needed for GTCA, but need be used to get explicit contour reconstructions in 2D TGDM applications. We include it here for convenience and completeness. In 2D, the only ambiguous case that needs special care is an ambiguous square, i.e., a square with two "inside" points in one diagonal and two "outside" points in the other diagonal. The correct tiling should separate the two "inside" points while connect the two "outside" ones if the "outside" points are 8-connected, and vice versa.

3.4 Topology Correction of Isosurfaces from General Data

As with other volumetric topology correction methods (except for the problematic global filtering approaches), the GTCA algorithm presented above works only on binary volumes (due to the digital topology principle it relies on). In practice, one often has to address the topology correction of isosurfaces computed from a gray-scale image or a floating-point valued volume. For example, many cortical surface reconstruction methods estimate the brain surfaces directly from the isosurface of a fuzzy membership function, a probability segmentation, or a preprocessed image intensity volume. In such cases, if we simply threshold the original data and then reconstruct the isosurface from the topology corrected binary volume, then the overall surface accuracy will be damaged. The resulting surface mesh will also suffer from the staircasing artifact due to the data binarization. Fortunately, a general isosurface topology correction algorithm can be easily designed by augmenting GTCA with a few extra steps. The new algorithm will produce a topology correct isosurface that is identical to the original isosurface except for some local changes at the handles being either cut or filled. The algorithm is presented below.

Algorithm 3.3 (Isosurface Topology Correction Algorithm)

1. Binarize the original gray-scale or floating-point valued volume I according to the specified isovalue v_{iso} to get a binary volume I_B.

2. Clean I_B to keep only the largest connected foreground component and fill its cavities if necessary. The result is denoted as I'_B.

3. Run GTCA on the volume I'_B to get the topology corrected volume I_T.

4. Compare the binary volumes I_B and I_T. If a foreground point in I_B is changed to background in I_T, then reduce the image value of this point in the original image I to a value below v_{iso} (any value below v_{iso} works). If a background point in I_B is changed to foreground in I_T, then we edit the image I at this

point to a value above v_{iso}. The edited image from I produces the final volume I'.

5. Compute the isosurface of I' using the CCMC algorithm with the original isovalue.

Since the new volume I' differs from the initial volume I only at local topological corrections made by GTCA, the new isosurface computed from I' will exactly agree with the original isosurface except at the locations of topology corrections. We note that it is critical to use the CCMC isosurface algorithm at the final step; otherwise, the surface topology will not match that of the volume, and new handles may appear. Note also that CCMC is a valid isosurface algorithm, producing the same accuracy as that of the standard MC algorithm. The only difference is that CCMC applies a digital connectivity rule in making choices between the ambiguous tilings, and the decision rule is consistent throughout the volume.

3.5 Results

3.5.1 Simple demonstration

We applied our algorithm to the piece of white matter shown in Fig. 3.12(a). Application of a foreground filter with $n = 18$ yields the object shown in Fig. 3.12(b), while a background filter with $\bar{n} = 6$ yields the object in Fig. 3.12(c). The foreground filter removed the handle by breaking it along a thin part, while the background filter filled the tunnel with a thin sheet. In both cases, the "cuts" are small and clearly not oriented in Cartesian directions. Figs. 3.12(d)–(h) depict the foreground cut (black) on a succession of slices through the object.

3.5.2 Brain volumes

The GTCA algorithm has been applied to over one hundred brain volumes (cf. Chapter 5) to perform topology correction on pre-segmented WM volumes, and it worked

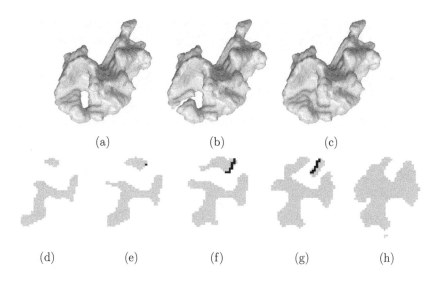

Figure 3.12: (a) A handle taken from an actual white matter volume. The result of using (b) a foreground filter and (c) a background filter. (d)-(h): Consecutive slices showing the cuts made by the foreground filter.

successfully every time. In this section, we present the results of extensive testing using 15 of these data sets to demonstrate the method's performance.

The typical WM volume size after partially cropping the background is $140 \times 200 \times 160$ voxels. Several versions of GTCA were applied to these data sets, including alternating foreground and background filters, foreground-only and background-only filters, alternate object connectivity definitions, and both ball-shaped and cross-shaped basic structuring elements. All filters produced the correct topology in the end, but their performances differed (see Tables 3.1–3.6).

The results shown in Tables 3.1–3.4 used 18-connectivity for the foreground, 6-connectivity for the background, and the 18-connected digital ball for the basic SE. The first row of the tables (under the headings) shows the original genus (number of handles) of the binarized white matter volumes, and the rows below show the genus after each filter stage until a zero genus is obtained in all image volumes. The leftmost entry in each row uses an abbreviated notation to indicate whether the filter is

Table 3.1: Genus, number of voxels changed and average number of changes per handle (ANCPH) of using a F-B sequence. $(n, \bar{n}) = (18, 6)$; SE = 18-ball.

Brain	S1	S2	S3	S4	S5	S6	S7	S8	S9	S10	S11	S12	S13	S14	S15
Original	724	955	1376	744	1031	776	562	886	688	825	986	597	1944	1280	801
f1	4	5	19	0	5	5	1	11	4	0	5	5	16	9	4
b1	0	0	1	-	2	0	0	1	0	-	0	1	0	0	0
f2	-	-	0	-	0	-	-	0	-	-	-	0	-	-	-
Changes	2144	2981	4028	1861	2990	1779	1491	2380	1953	2029	2549	1493	5954	3514	2096
ANCPH	2.96	3.12	2.93	2.50	2.90	2.29	2.65	2.69	2.84	2.46	2.58	2.50	3.06	2.74	2.62

Table 3.2: Genus, number of voxels changed and average number of changes per handle (ANCPH) of using a B-F sequence. $(n, \bar{n}) = (18, 6)$; SE = 18-ball.

Brain	S1	S2	S3	S4	S5	S6	S7	S8	S9	S10	S11	S12	S13	S14	S15
Original	724	955	1376	744	1031	776	562	886	688	825	986	597	1944	1280	801
b1	46	31	31	39	31	24	16	33	26	23	20	17	57	36	20
f1	0	0	0	0	1	0	0	1	0	0	0	0	0	0	0
b2	-	-	-	-	1	-	-	0	-	-	-	-	-	-	-
f2	-	-	-	-	0	-	-	-	-	-	-	-	-	-	-
Changes	1371	1915	2526	1434	1984	1352	1049	1576	1257	1493	1717	1051	3812	2477	1498
ANCPH	1.89	2.00	1.84	1.93	1.92	1.74	1.87	1.78	1.83	1.81	1.74	1.76	1.96	1.93	1.87

a foreground (f) or background (b) filter and the scale of the structuring element. For example, the notation "f2" means foreground filter with structuring element size 2 (the basic SE dilated by itself once) and "b3" means background filter with structuring element size 3. The second to last row shows the number of voxels changed in the final topologically correct volumes as compared with the original ones. The last row shows the *average number of voxels changed per handle* (ANCPH), which is the ratio of the total number of voxels changed to the genus of the original volume.

Tables 3.1 and 3.2 show the results from alternating sequences of foreground and background filters with increasing scale. Comparing the results of the two tables, we see that there are always fewer voxels changed (better ANCPH) when the background filter is applied first. The reason for this is that the background filter assumes

Table 3.3: Genus, number of voxels changed and average number of changes per handle (ANCPH) of using F-filters only. $(n, \bar{n}) = (18, 6)$; SE = 18-ball.

Brain	S1	S2	S3	S4	S5	S6	S7	S8	S9	S10	S11	S12	S13	S14	S15
Original	724	955	1376	744	1031	776	562	886	688	825	986	597	1944	1280	801
f1	4	5	19	0	5	5	1	11	4	0	5	5	16	9	4
f2	0	0	0	0	0	0	0	0	0	-	1	0	0	0	0
f3	-	-	-	-	-	-	-	-	-	-	0	-	-	-	-
Changes	2218	3058	4755	1861	3050	1893	1504	2705	2083	2029	2879	1538	6421	3830	2234
ANCPH	3.06	3.20	3.46	2.50	2.96	2.44	2.68	3.05	3.03	2.46	2.92	2.58	3.30	2.99	2.79

Table 3.4: Genus, number of voxels changed and average number of changes per handle (ANCPH) of using B-filters only. $(n, \bar{n}) = (18, 6)$; SE = 18-ball.

Brain	S1	S2	S3	S4	S5	S6	S7	S8	S9	S10	S11	S12	S13	S14	S15
Original	724	955	1376	744	1031	776	562	886	688	825	986	597	1944	1280	801
b1	46	31	31	39	31	24	16	33	26	23	20	17	57	36	20
b2	7	7	3	6	6	1	2	6	4	5	6	3	9	6	5
b3	0	1	0	0	0	0	0	1	0	0	1	0	3	1	1
b4	-	0	-	-	-	-	-	0	-	-	0	-	0	0	0
Changes	1951	2827	3319	1777	2284	1768	1287	2181	1617	1785	1962	1395	4836	2907	2101
ANCPH	2.69	2.96	2.41	2.39	2.22	2.28	2.29	2.46	2.35	2.16	1.99	2.34	2.49	2.27	2.62

6-connectivity while the foreground assumes 18-connectivity. As a result, narrower "swaths" can be used to fill tunnels in the background. On the other hand, the foreground filter yields a faster *initial* reduction in the genus, which shows that the original white matter segmentations have more thin handles than small tunnels. As shown in the tables, the ratio of the number of voxels changed to the genus of the original volume is around 2.8 for the F-B sequence and less than 2 for the B-F sequence. It should be noted that the quality of the initial segmentation has a substantial impact on ANCPH. Therefore, although our results are comparable to those in [143, 144] this does not allow us to conclude that the algorithms are comparable. A direct comparison on the same data is needed.

Tables 3.3 and 3.4 show the results arising from the application of only one type of

Table 3.5: Genus, number of voxels changed and average number of changes per handle (ANCPH) of using a B-F sequence. $(n, \bar{n}) = (18, 6)$, SE = 6-cross.

Brain	S1	S2	S3	S4	S5	S6	S7	S8	S9	S10	S11	S12	S13	S14	S15
Original	724	955	1376	744	1031	776	562	886	688	825	986	597	1944	1280	801
b1	130	166	144	98	108	94	66	103	94	108	103	77	249	169	85
f1	2	9	12	4	3	3	7	11	6	3	6	5	8	8	7
b2	1	4	5	3	1	0	3	5	2	0	3	1	3	3	5
f2	0	0	1	0	1	-	0	0	0	-	0	0	0	0	0
b3	-	-	0	-	0	-	-	-	-	-	-	-	-	-	-
Changes	1270	1714	2335	1346	1782	1238	972	1497	1126	1296	1573	993	3734	2136	1283
ANCPH	1.75	1.79	1.70	1.81	1.73	1.60	1.73	1.69	1.64	1.57	1.60	1.66	1.92	1.67	1.60

Table 3.6: Genus, number of voxels changed and average number of changes per handle (ANCPH) of using a F-B sequence $(n, \bar{n}) = (26, 6)$; SE = 18-ball.

Brain	S1	S2	S3	S4	S5	S6	S7	S8	S9	S10	S11	S12	S13	S14	S15
Original	1049	1354	2008	1075	1522	1132	863	1313	979	1201	1438	854	2726	1843	1186
f1	12	11	35	0	13	12	2	14	8	5	12	9	21	11	12
b1	1	0	1	-	2	0	0	2	0	0	0	1	1	0	0
f2	0	-	0	-	0	-	-	0	-	-	-	0	0	-	-
Changes	3046	4004	5559	2612	4080	2541	2115	3240	2642	2817	3516	2051	8221	4655	2859
ANCPH	2.90	2.96	2.77	2.43	2.68	2.24	2.45	2.47	2.70	2.34	2.44	2.40	3.02	2.52	2.41

filter, foreground or background, respectively. These tables verify that our algorithm can achieve a topologically correct result by either cutting handles or filling tunnels exclusively. It is also observed that the background filters yield overall fewer changes to the volume than the foreground filters. Once again this can be attributed to the fact that the background filters assume 6-connectivity rather than 18-connectivity. Comparing these tables to Tables 3.1 and 3.2 also shows that the topological correction with the smallest modification to the volume is achieved by alternating background and foreground filters. This process guarantees that a topological defect is corrected at the smallest possible scale.

Table 3.5 shows the results of using the 3D cross as the basic SE instead of the 18-ball. Again, the correct topology is achieved for each data set. Comparing this

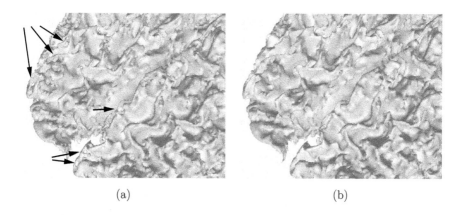

(a)	(b)

Figure 3.13: Cortical surfaces obtained (a) before and (b) after topology correction.

result to that in Table 3.2 reveals that the cross has better performance as measured by the total number of voxels changed. This is attributed to the fact that the cross has finer structure than the ball, so defects can be corrected at even finer scales. The tradeoff is that the cross requires five scales instead of four — and therefore more computation time — in order to guarantee topological correctness of all 15 volumes.

Table 3.6 shows the result from application of 26-connectivity to the foreground and 6-connectivity to the background. As expected, GTCA successfully corrects the topology of all 15 brain volumes. Comparison with Table 3.1, however, shows that it does not perform as well as the (18,6) topological pair, as measured by the number of voxels changed in the final volume. It is also interesting to note that use of 26-connectivity yields a much larger genus in the *original* volume than does use of 18-connectivity. These facts taken together suggest that use of (18,6) connectivity rather than (26,6) connectivity will produce a more delicate topological correction.

3.5.3   Visualization and computation

Fig. 3.13 shows one part of a WM/GM surface before and after topology correction using a background-foreground sequence with 6 connectivity for the background and 18-connectivity for the foreground. The basic structuring element used in this experiment is the 18-ball. All handles seen in panel (a) are clearly removed in panel (b).

The processing time of GTCA depends on the total number of foreground/background filters required. For the results shown in Tables 3.1–3.6, each filter took less than 30 seconds on a 2.2 GHz Intel Pentium4 PC running a Linux operating system, and the total processing time for each brain volume took less than 2 minutes.

3.6 Discussion

We have experimentally shown that our topology correction algorithm works successfully on brain volumes having large numbers of handles. Furthermore, it works successfully with different choices of connectivity rules, different filtering sequences, and different structuring elements. It is clear from the theory that it will always produce a topologically correct final volume; however, we make no claim that our result is optimal by any criteria. Instead, our approach can be considered to be a (presumably) sub-optimal solution to the goal of producing a topologically correct object by making the fewest number of changes to the voxels in the original volume.

It might be asked whether the criterion of making the fewest number of changes to the original volume is a sensible one, especially in the practical application of cortical surface reconstruction. The primary rationale behind this criterion is that topology defects are caused by image noise, and are primarily of a fine scale. Our strategy to alternate between foreground and background, then go from fine to coarse scales acknowledges the fact that such noise can either "add" or "remove" parts of the object and that noise can sometimes group together to form larger defects. But this focus and strategy does not necessarily make changes that are concordant with the actual anatomy. For example, a problem we have encountered in the practical application of GTCA is that it sometimes cause a undesired cut at the temporal lobe of the brain cortex. The reason is that at the temporal lobe, the WM tends to be misclassified as GM, which often results in a thin handle at a temporal lobe gyrus. If a foreground-background sequence is used, the handle tends to be cut in the first foreground filtering pass, while it is desirable to fill in the tunnel created by the misclassification. Currently, we address this problem by always applying the background filter first, and find that it helps producing the desired topology correction most of the times. But to fully address this problem, it is necessary to incorporate additional anatomical knowledge into the decision about how a handle should be removed.

As another example, suppose two opposing banks of a sulcus were wrongly "bridged". The two possible corrections to this topological defect are to remove the bridge or to fill the entire sulcus. If the sulcus were very narrow and the bridge were very thick, then it is possible that our algorithm would erroneously fill the sulcus. Fortunately, the above situation is unlikely to exist when correcting the white matter volume, since the sulcal separation includes both the sulcal gap itself and both sulcal banks comprising cortical gray matter. Therefore, it is unlikely that such bridges will exist, assuming a good segmentation algorithm is used. Furthermore, it is much more likely that the scale of any such bridge will be smaller than the scale of the sulcus. In this case, the bridge will be cut first and the correct result will be achieved regardless of the order of background and foreground alternation. On the other hand, if our algorithm were applied to a segmentation comprising both the gray matter and white matter, then an erroneous sulcal filling is more likely. Thus, it is important for the production of anatomically correct results that a good segmentation algorithm be used, and our correction algorithm is applied on the white matter segmentation.

3.7 Summary

In this chapter, we developed and evaluated GTCA, an automatic method to remove handles in 3D digital images. GTCA is fundamentally based on the theory of digital topology and uses results from mathematical morphology, implicit surface tiling, and graph theory. The method has been shown to work very well on 15 magnetic resonance segmented volumes and has been successfully applied on over one hundred MR brain volumes. We expect GTCA to be a useful automated tool that can help the processing of large numbers of brain data sets for brain geometric and functional analysis studies across populations.

84

Chapter 4

Topology-preserving Geometric Deformable Model

The GTCA and other topology correction methods can be used to get a topologically correct boundary reconstruction from an initial image segmentation having the
wrong topology. But these methods still have limitations. First, they cannot be used
as an image segmentation method by themselves. Second, it is difficult to incorporate additional image information or prior object shape knowledge into the topology
correction procedure. Thus, these methods are typically used as one processing step
in a complete medical image segmentation system [65, 140]. In Chapter 5, we will
show the development of one such system, which successfully combines the GTCA
method with a new geometric deformable model in order to get accurate and topologically correct brain cortex segmentations. The new geometric deformable model
is the topic of the present chapter. Before we go on to present the details, we first
briefly summarize the method and its motivation, and introduce the organization of
this chapter.

The development of the new geometric deformable model method aims to combine
the topology preserving properties of PDMs with the parameterization free, implicit
representation of traditional GDMs. The new deformable model guarantees that the
final contour (curve or surface) has the prescribed model topology, and has a valid
manifold structure without any self-intersection. The development starts with the

design of a *topology-preserving level set method* (TLSM). In contrast to the standard level set method where no control of the evolving contour topology ever exists, TLSM guarantees that the evolving implicit contour has exactly the same topology as the initial one. TLSM also inherits the property of standard level set method that contour self-intersections cannot occur. TLSM can be used with any existing 2D or 3D geometric deformable model, regardless of the internal or external force definition, yielding the new geometric deformable model method, which we will refer to as *topology-preserving geometric deformable model* (TGDM). We note that TGDM maintains the sub-pixel interpolation and boundary regularization properties of traditional geometric deformable models, which distinguishes our method from the topology-preserving region growing method of Mangin et al. [13].

The remainder of this chapter is organized as follows. We start with an overview of the basic principles underlying this new deformable model in Section 4.1, especially the *digital embedding* of the implicit contour topology. We then present our topology-preserving narrow band algorithm in Section 4.2. To better understand the convergence properties of the new TLSM algorithm, we present in Section 4.3 an interpretation of this algorithm as a constrained gradient descent algorithm in the special case of the geodesic deformable model. Experimental results on both 2D and 3D phantoms and real data are shown in Section 4.4 to demonstrate the behavior and advantages of the new TGDMs, which also serve as an illustration for their potential applications. Section 4.5 discusses the results, and gives more details on the connections between previous work and our approach. Finally, we summarize the chapter in Section 4.6.

4.1   Overview of Basic Principles

4.1.1   Digital embedding of topology

Although geometric deformable models are formulated on the continuum, in practice they are always implemented on a digital domain — i.e., on a lattice of grid points connected by grid cells ("cubes" as in the Marching Cubes algorithm). Without restrictions on their functional form, there are, in general, an infinite number of contours having the same sampled level set function. Since these contours can have different numbers of components with different topologies, it is clear that it is generally impossible to recover the "true" topology of an arbitrary implicit contour from samples of its level set function. Therefore, in order to give meaning to the idea of "preserving topology" in a geometric deformable model, we must adopt certain conventions about the nature of the implied contour given its sampled level set function. The convention we describe below addresses the following two broad ambiguities. First, a continuous implicit contour might be entirely contained in one grid cell or it might intersect a cell boundary any number of times. These phenomena basically describe types of high frequency behavior not captured by the digital samples. Second, even if the contour is slowly varying, there might still be ambiguities as to how a cell is actually partitioned by a contour. This ambiguity is directly tied to the classical problems of ambiguous cubes and faces in isocontour algorithms as introduced in Chapter 2.

To resolve these topological ambiguities, in this book we adopt a digital interpretation of the implicit contour topology. First, we assume that the zero level set changes sufficiently slowly that it can only pass between neighboring grid points once at most. In adopting this assumption, we are thereby ignoring topological details of the zero level set that cannot be recovered under a given discretization of the computational domain. As shown in Fig. 4.1, this assumption ties the topology of the zero level set with that of the digital object it encircles. More specifically, assuming that Φ denotes the embedding level set function as introduced in Chapter 2, we classify grid points for which $\Phi < 0$ as *inside* the zero level set, and for which $\Phi > 0$ as *outside*. Then the *digital object* consists of all the *inside* points. To avoid further ambiguity, we also adopt the convention that grid points for which $\Phi = 0$ are considered to be inside the zero level set.

The second ambiguity is resolved by specifying a pair of consistent connectivity rules for the digital object (i.e., the foreground) and its background. For example, in 2D we might choose the object to be 4-connected, in which case the background must be 8-connected (see Chapter 2 for the definition of digital connectivities in both

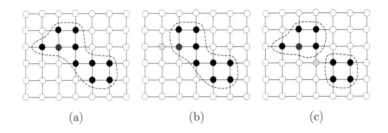

Figure 4.1: Topology equivalence of the embedded contour and the digital object it defines on the discrete grid: 4-connectivity for dark points and 8-connectivity for others. (a) Original contour. (b) The contour passes over a simple point. (c) The contour splits at a non-simple point.

2D and 3D). Alternatively, we could choose the foreground to be 8-connected and the background to be 4-connected. As introduced before, the consistent connectivity rules in 3D are (6,18), (6,26), (18,6), and (26,6), where the first number in each pair is the foreground connectivity and the second number is the background connectivity. These rules prevent topological anomalies that might, for example, allow a closed path in the background to pass through a simple connected foreground component.

From now on, we always treat the topology of the zero level set to be equivalent to the topology of the boundary of the digital object it defines. This equivalence makes sense since we can view the zero level set contour as a homeomorphic deformation of the discrete object boundary drawn on the grid. We refer to this equivalence as the *digital embedding* of the zero level set topology.

4.1.2 Topology preservation

The principle of digital embedding simplifies the topology preservation problem. Since the digital object is defined by thresholding the level set function at the zero isovalue, it is clear that the topology of the implicit contour can change only if the level set function changes sign at a grid point,[8] which corresponds to a point moving from inside the digital object to the background or vice versa.

---

[8]Note that by our convention a sign change also happens if a zero value becomes positive or vice versa.

From the above discussion, we conclude that it is only necessary to be concerned about topological changes when the level set function is going to change sign. But switching a grid point from background to foreground (or vice versa) does not necessarily change the object's topology. In fact, from the theory of digital topology (see review in Chapter 2), we find that the topology of the digital object will *not* change if the grid point under consideration is a *simple point* [129, 131, 132, 151], as illustrated in Fig. 4.1(b). On the other hand, if the grid point is not a simple point, as illustrated in Fig. 4.1(c), then the digital object's topology *will* change. Now our entire strategy becomes clear. During the evolution of the level set function, we monitor the level set function for potential sign changes. If the sign is scheduled to change at a simple point, then it is allowed; but, sign changes at non-simple points are not allowed. This prevents topology changes of the underlying digital object and of the implicit zero level set as well. We note that the deforming implicit contour need not "get stuck" at a non-simple point, since the point can become simple after additional evolution of the contour; several examples of this type of behavior are shown in Section 4.4.

There are two key observations to make about this overall approach. First, since it is necessary to explicitly monitor the sign of the level set function at each grid point, a time-explicit implementation is required. The standard narrow band approach is both time-explicit and computationally fast, so it represents an ideal framework for our algorithm. Second, we observe that the topology of the implicit contour is determined by the sign of the level set function, not its particular value. Therefore, the level set function is free to change its value in order to refine the position of the implicit contour at a *subpixel resolution*. In particular, despite the use of digital topology principles to control topology, the accuracy of the deformable model itself is still at the same subpixel level that is possible with standard geometric deformable models. A similar situation was observed in the design of the isosurface topology correction algorithm in Chapter 3.

4.1.3   Explicit contour topology

We have now presented the basic notions describing how to relate the topology of the implicit contour to the discrete level set function and how to evolve the level set function in order to preserve topology. It is also important that we be able to *reconstruct* an explicit contour of the zero level set — a curve in 2D and a surface in 3D — and to guarantee that this reconstructed contour has the same topology as the digital object's boundary.

In Section 3.3 of Chapter 3, we presented the CCMC and the CCMS isocontour algorithms, and mentioned that their design was exactly aimed to address the need to get topologically correct isocontour reconstructions that are consistent with the digital topology embedding principle. Thus, we can apply the CCMS or the CCMC algorithm to get an explicit representation of the implicit contour from the embedding level set function. It is this explicit contour that we visualize (see Results), and that we use to characterize the topology of the evolving geometric deformable model.

As introduced in Chapter 2, the topology of a given distinct contour can be summarized using its Euler characteristics or Euler number χ, which can be computed from (2.13) (note that N_F is always zero for a 2D curve). Thus, in principle, it is possible to *monitor* topological changes that are taking place during evolution of the level set function by counting the number of distinct contours and evaluating their Euler characteristics. The result of this computation cannot be used to *control* the topology since it is a global property of the contour(s), but it can be used to *verify* that a topology preserving mechanism is actually working properly. We used this computation in our experiments (see Results section) to verify that both the evolving contour and the final contour had the correct topology. It is not necessary, however, to compute the Euler characteristics in order to run TGDM.

4.2   Topology-preserving Narrow Band Algorithm

In this section, we present the implementation of TLSM. The implementation consists of a subtle but important modification to the standard narrow band algorithm

(Algorithm 2.1 in Chapter 2), which keeps the topology of the contour defined by the zero level set unchanged during the entire evolution. One important issue regarding the convergence properties of geometric deformable models implemented using TLSM will be considered in the next section.

As introduced in Chapter 2, the narrow band method is designed to efficiently solve the time-dependent PDE governing the deformation of the level set function, (2.5) and (2.10), or its numerically discretized counterpart, (2.12). For convenience, we repeat (2.12) here:

$$\Phi(\mathbf{x}_i, t_{m+1}) = \Phi(\mathbf{x}_i, t_m) + \Delta t \Delta \Phi(\mathbf{x}_i, t_m), \tag{4.1}$$

where $\Phi(\cdot, \cdot)$ denotes the discretized level set function. Also, t_m and t_{m+1} denote two consecutive discrete time steps, $\Delta t = t_{m+1} - t_m$ is the time-step size, $\mathbf{x}_i$ denotes a generic grid point, and $\Delta \Phi$ is the upwind numerical approximation to the force terms in the original level set PDE, (2.10).

In the following algorithm, it is convenient to store a binary-valued indicator function $B(\cdot)$, defined on the digital grid. For a grid point $\mathbf{x}_i$, $B(\mathbf{x}_i)$ equals 1 if $\Phi(\mathbf{x}_i, t_m) \leq 0$, and equals 0 otherwise, where t_m is the last time the point $\mathbf{x}_i$ is visited. The array $B(\cdot)$ is initialized using $\Phi(\cdot, 0)$, and is updated whenever the level set function Φ undergoes a sign change at a grid point $\mathbf{x}_i$. The sign change is computed using the following sign function definition, which reflects our convention that a zero valued grid point belongs to the interior of the zero level set:

$$\text{sign}(x) = \begin{cases} 1, & \text{if } x \leq 0; \\ -1, & \text{if } x > 0. \end{cases} \tag{4.2}$$

The TLSM algorithm is summarized below. Here, $\mathbf{x}_i$ is used to denote a general grid point and $\mathbf{y}_i$ denotes a narrow band point.

Algorithm 4.1 (Topology-preserving Level Set Method)

1. *Initialize* — Set $m = 0$ and $t_m = 0$. Initialize $\Phi(\cdot, 0)$ to be the signed distance function of the initial contour. Initialize the binary indicator function B.

2. *Build the Narrow Band* — Find all grid points $\mathbf{y}_i, i \in \{1, \ldots, Q\}$ such that $|\Phi(\mathbf{y}_i, t_m)| < W_{\mathrm{nb}}$, where W_{nb} is the user-specified narrow band width, and Q denotes the total number of narrow band points.

3. *Update* — For $i = 1, \cdots, Q$, compute the level set function at the narrow band point $\mathbf{y}_i$ at time $t_{m+1} = t_m + \Delta t$ by:

   (a) Using (4.1), compute $\Phi_{\mathrm{temp}}(\mathbf{y}_i) = \Phi(\mathbf{y}_i, t_m) + \Delta t \Delta \Phi(\mathbf{y}_i, t_m)$.

   (b) If $\mathrm{sign}(\Phi_{\mathrm{temp}}(\mathbf{y}_i)) = \mathrm{sign}(\Phi(\mathbf{y}_i, t_m))$, then set $\Phi(\mathbf{y}_i, t_{m+1}) = \Phi_{\mathrm{temp}}(\mathbf{y}_i)$, keep $B(\mathbf{y}_i)$ unchanged, and go to Step 3(f). Otherwise continue to Step 3(c).

   (c) Test whether $\mathbf{y}_i$ is a simple point by computing two topological numbers $T_n(\mathbf{y}_i, X)$ and $T_{\bar{n}}(\mathbf{y}_i, \bar{X})$ (cf. Chapter 2), where $(n, \bar{n})$ is the chosen digital connectivity pair, $X = \{\,\mathbf{x}_i \mid B(\mathbf{x}_i) = 1\,\}$, and $\bar{X} = \{\,\mathbf{x}_i \mid B(\mathbf{x}_i) = 0\,\}$.

   (d) If the point is simple — i.e., $T_n(\mathbf{y}_i, X) = T_{\bar{n}}(\mathbf{y}_i, \bar{X}) = 1$ — then set $\Phi(\mathbf{y}_i, t_{m+1}) = \Phi_{\mathrm{temp}}(\mathbf{y}_i)$, $B(\mathbf{y}_i) = (B(\mathbf{y}_i) + 1) \bmod 2$, and go to Step 3(f). Otherwise continue to Step 3(e).

   (e) Point $\mathbf{y}_i$ is not simple. To preserve the topology, we do not allow the sign change and set $\Phi(\mathbf{y}_i, t_{m+1}) = \epsilon \cdot \mathrm{sign}(\Phi(\mathbf{y}_i, t_m))$, where ϵ is a small positive number. Note that $B(\mathbf{y}_i)$ remains unchanged.

   (f) Increase i. If $i > Q$, go to Step 4.

4. *Reinitialize* — If the zero level set of $\Phi(\cdot, t_{m+1})$ is near the boundary of the current narrow band, reinitialize $\Phi(\cdot, t_{m+1})$ to be the signed distance function of its zero level set.

5. *Convergence Test* — Test whether the zero level set has stopped moving. If yes, stop; otherwise, set $m = m + 1$. If reinitialization was performed in Step 4, then go back to Step 2 to rebuild the narrow band; otherwise, go back to Step 3. ∎

After the level set iterations have converged, we extract the final contour using the CCMS (2D) or CCMC (3D) algorithm presented in Section 3.3 of Chapter 3. As stated there, the contour location is computed by linear interpolation of the level set function, but the tiling for the ambiguous cases is selected based on the chosen digital connectivity pair. If the level set function value is exactly zero at a grid point, it is explicitly adjusted before interpolation to prevent singularities in the resulting contour (cf. Chapter 2). Since we consider zero-valued points to be inside points, i.e., as negative distance points, we set a zero function value to some small negative value, say $-\epsilon$.

Compared with Algorithm 2.1, the TLSM algorithm differs only in the Update step, which performs a simple point criterion check whenever the level set function is scheduled to change sign at a grid point. The sign change is prohibited if the point is not a simple point, and the evolution of the level set function at that point is limited. One might ask how this limiting operation would affect the convergence property of the new model. We show in the next section that the above algorithm is a direct analog of the gradient-descent-with-bending algorithm in the literature of constrained optimization [153], and thus is guaranteed to converge to a constrained optimum.

We would like to point out that there can be some arbitrariness in the specific result of the algorithm depending on the order in which the points are visited in the narrow band. This situation is also present in skeletonization algorithms where the result depends on the order of simple point removal [154]. The problem is not as significant here as in skeletonization, however, since the overall motion of the deforming contour is controlled by the internal and external forces. The simple point criterion only takes effect at locations where topological changes are otherwise going to occur, and these locations ordinarily comprise a very small portion of the overall contour. Still, we have compared the results of two different orderings for visiting the narrow band points. In one case we ordered the points by the magnitude of their external force, and in the other case by a natural ordering that "rasters" through the coordinates of the points. The difference was trivial, and did not favor either approach. In the experiments reported herein, we visit the narrow band points by the natural "raster" ordering of their coordinates.

4.3 Convergence Analysis

To analyze the convergence property of TLSM-based geometric deformable models (i.e., a TGDM), we focus on the case where the model is derived from an energy minimization framework, for example, the geodesic deformable model. In the original formulation of the geodesic deformable model (cf. Section 2.3.2 and (2.7) in Chapter 2), the energy to be minimized is defined as a functional on the family of explicitly parameterized contours. The level set evolution equation is then derived by applying the level set method. By adopting the techniques presented in [123, 155], we can derive the evolution equation of the geodesic deformable model directly from an energy functional defined on the level set function itself. We can then show that the corresponding TGDM algorithm in this case is a constrained gradient descent algorithm, and is guaranteed to converge to a constrained optimal point of the energy functional.

Assume that the deformable contour is embedded as the zero level set of a Lipschitz-continuous level set function $\Phi(\mathbf{x}), \mathbf{x} \in \Omega$ where $\Omega \subset \mathcal{R}^2$ (resp. $\mathcal{R}^3$). Then, it can be proved by the co-area formula [156] that the length (resp. area) of the zero level set of Φ is given by:

$$L(\Phi) = \int_\Omega \delta(\Phi(\mathbf{x}))|\nabla\Phi(\mathbf{x})|d\mathbf{x},$$

where $\delta(\cdot)$ is the one-dimensional Dirac delta function. Similarly, the weighted length or area L_g under an image derived metric $g(\mathbf{x})$ can be rewritten as

$$L_g(\Phi) = \int_\Omega \delta(\Phi(\mathbf{x}))|\nabla\Phi(\mathbf{x})|gd\mathbf{x}.$$

To make the equations shorter, in the following derivation we omit the function argument $\mathbf{x}$ when there is no potential for confusion.

The Frechet derivative of L_g with respect to $\Phi(\mathbf{x})$ in the direction $h(\mathbf{x})$, which is denoted by $dL_g(\Phi, h)$, can be computed as

$$dL_g(\Phi, h) = \int_\Omega h\delta'(\Phi)|\nabla\Phi|gd\mathbf{x} + \int_\Omega \delta(\Phi)g\frac{\nabla\Phi \cdot \nabla h}{|\nabla\Phi|}d\mathbf{x},$$

where $\delta'(\cdot)$ denotes the first derivative of the delta function.

Applying Green's formula [119] to the second term yields

$$dL_g(\Phi, h) = \int_\Omega h\delta'(\Phi)|\nabla\Phi|gd\mathbf{x} + \oint_{\partial\Omega} h\delta(\Phi)g\frac{\nabla\Phi \cdot \vec{N}}{|\nabla\Phi|}ds - \int_\Omega h\nabla \cdot (\delta(\Phi)g\frac{\nabla\Phi}{|\nabla\Phi|})d\mathbf{x},$$

where $\nabla\cdot$ is the divergence operator, $\vec{N}$ is the outward-pointing normal vector to the boundary, and ds is a differential element on the boundary.

Since $\nabla\Phi \cdot \vec{N} = \partial\Phi/\partial\vec{N}$ and

$$\nabla \cdot (\delta(\Phi)g\frac{\nabla\Phi}{|\nabla\Phi|}) = g\delta'(\Phi)|\nabla\Phi| + \delta(\Phi)\nabla \cdot (g\frac{\nabla\Phi}{|\nabla\Phi|}),$$

under the natural boundary condition $\partial\Phi/\partial\vec{N} = 0$ we get

$$
\begin{aligned}
dL_g(\Phi, h) &= -\int_\Omega \delta(\Phi)\nabla \cdot (g\frac{\nabla\Phi}{|\nabla\Phi|})h d\mathbf{x} \\
&= <-\delta(\Phi)\nabla \cdot (g\frac{\nabla\Phi}{|\nabla\Phi|}), h>,
\end{aligned}
$$

where $< \cdot, \cdot >$ denotes inner product in the L^2 sense. From the Schwartz inequality [119], it is clear that the direction that reduces the energy functional L_g most rapidly — that is, the steepest descent direction h_s — is given by

$$h_s = \delta(\Phi)\nabla \cdot (g\frac{\nabla\Phi}{|\nabla\Phi|}) = \delta(\Phi)\left\{\frac{\nabla g \cdot \nabla\Phi}{|\nabla\Phi|} + g\nabla \cdot (\frac{\nabla\Phi}{|\nabla\Phi|})\right\},$$

where the second equality follows from a vector calculus identity. Thus, starting from an initial estimate $\Phi(\mathbf{x}, 0)$, the gradient descent algorithm with an infinitesimal time step δt gives the level set evolution equation as

$$\frac{\partial\Phi(\mathbf{x}, t)}{\partial t} = h_s(\mathbf{x}) = \delta(\Phi(\mathbf{x}, t))\left\{\frac{\nabla g(\mathbf{x}) \cdot \nabla\Phi(\mathbf{x}, t)}{|\nabla\Phi(\mathbf{x}, t)|} + g(\mathbf{x})\nabla \cdot (\frac{\nabla\Phi(\mathbf{x}, t)}{|\nabla\Phi(\mathbf{x}, t)|})\right\}, \quad (4.3)$$

such that the family of level set functions $\Phi(\cdot, t)$ will converge to the (local) minimum of the energy functional L_g as t goes to infinity.

We can see that the only difference between (2.9) and (4.3) is that the scale factor $\delta(\Phi(\mathbf{x}, t))$ in (4.3) is replaced by $|\nabla\Phi(\mathbf{x}, t)|$ in (2.9), which corresponds to extending the evolution equation to all the level sets of Φ [155]. Since the energy functional L_g depends only on the zero level set of Φ, we note that (2.9) also gives a steepest descent minimization of L_g.

When topology preservation is required, the gradient descent process must be constrained to the admissible set (or feasible domain) of level set functions that satisfy the topology constraint. In our case, this feasible domain comprises level set functions whose zero level sets share the prescribed model topology. From an optimization viewpoint, we can think of a single step of the gradient descent algorithm as a modification of the entire level set function in order to produce a new level set function. If that new function were outside of the feasible domain (i.e., its zero level set did not have the correct topology), then one possible modification to the algorithm would be to reduce the step size until the modified function remained in the feasible domain. Unfortunately, this simple strategy has been shown in the literature on constrained optimization to suffer from the "jamming" effect and non-convergence [153, 157]. To avoid the jamming effect (and thereby to guarantee convergence), McCormick [153] proposed the *constrained gradient descent with bending* algorithm. The key idea is that instead of reducing the whole step size, which is equivalent to multiplying the descent vector by a small constant, only that component of the descent vector which leads outside the feasible domain should be reduced (or truncated) while the other components should keep the usual step size. This strategy has been shown to avoid the jamming effect and to always converge to a constrained stationary point, i.e., a Kuhn-Tucker point [157].

Our TGDM algorithm is an adaptation of McCormick's approach. To see this, we note that an individual component of the gradient descent vector in the geodesic deformable model is exactly the force function evaluated at an individual grid point. Those components that lead to a violation of the topology constraint, and therefore would move the whole level set function out of the feasible domain, can be determined by the simple point criterion. Step 3(e) in the topology-preserving narrow band algorithm thus corresponds to the truncating of the component of the gradient descending vector that would lead to movement out of the feasible domain; the other components remain unchanged. This is exactly the *bending* of the gradient descent direction as described in [153].

As pointed out previously, there can be some arbitrariness in the specific result of the algorithm depending on the order in which the grid points are visited in the narrow band. This arbitrariness reflects the fact that the feasible domain of the topology-constrained minimization problem is non-convex. As a result, at a concave corner of the feasible domain, there can be more than one possible direction to bend the original gradient descent vector. Which direction the bending actually occurs depends on the order in which the grid points are visited.

We note that as the unconstrained model can only be guaranteed to converge to a local optimum depending on the initialization, the TGDM may also only converge to a constrained local optimum. We also note that in a general geometric deformable model where the evolution equation does not come from an energy minimization formulation, the above optimality and convergence analysis does not apply. But from our experience and as demonstrated in the presented experiment results, the TGDM algorithm shares the same convergence property as its non-constrained counterpart.

4.4 Results

In this section, we present several experiments which apply the new topology-preserving geometric deformable models in 2D and 3D. Since the new models can be obtained from existing geometric deformable models by applying the TLSM narrow band implementation, we refer to the original models without topology constraint (implemented by the standard narrow band algorithm) as *standard geometric deformable models* (SGDMs) and the corresponding (i.e., with the same set of force terms) topology-preserving models as *topology-preserving geometric deformable models* TGDMs. When a parametric deformable model with a similar set of force terms is also compared, it will be referred to as the *parametric deformable model* (PDM). Note that for the TGDM, the CCMS or CCMC algorithm must be used in order to correctly extract the final curves or surfaces from the level set function. The SGDM, on the other hand, requires a standard isocontour algorithm, preferably one that uses face saddle points in 2D and both face and body saddle points in 3D [137]. In the following experiments, we choose $(n, \bar{n}) = (4, 8)$ as the pair of 2D digital connectivities and $(n, \bar{n}) = (18, 6)$ for 3D.

4.4.1 2D experiments

Fig. 4.2 shows a 2D example that compares the behavior of PDM, SGDM, and TGDM. All three models apply a curvature force as the smoothing internal force

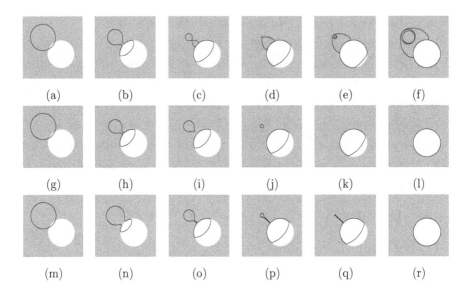

Figure 4.2: A 2D phantom illustrating the self-intersection problem of PDM. (a)–(f): propagation of the PDM contour at several time steps; (g)–(l): evolution of the SGDM contour; (m)–(r): evolution of the TGDM model.

and a region force that expands inside the white circular cell and contracts outside. The top row of Fig. 4.2 shows the propagation of the PDM contour at several time steps starting from the initialization shown in Fig. 4.2(a). The curve intersects with itself and then goes unstable because the normal direction gets flipped over after the curve self-intersects and the region force begins to push the curve in the wrong direction. The SGDM curve (the middle row) changes topology twice, first splitting in Fig. 4.2(i) and then losing one curve in Fig. 4.2(k). On the other hand, the TGDM curve maintains the same topology throughout its evolution and does not suffer from the self-intersection problem. It is apparent that in this case the SGDM and the TGDM produced the same final contour.

The second 2D experiment, shown in Fig. 4.3, used the same phantom but a different initialization. A variation of the geodesic deformable contour model of (2.9) was used as the SGDM model, where an additional expansion force $cg(\mathbf{x})|\nabla\Phi(\mathbf{x}, t)|$ (with

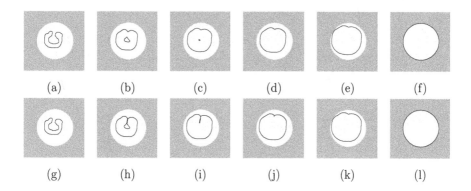

(a) (b) (c) (d) (e) (f)

(g) (h) (i) (j) (k) (l)

Figure 4.3: Illustration of TGDM reaching the same global optimum as SGDM. (a)–(f): SGDM result; (g)–(l): TGDM result.

c constant) was added to increase the speed of convergence [46]. The final contour thus corresponds to the solution of the geodesic energy minimization problem. The corresponding TGDM model was derived from the SGDM by imposing the topology-preserving constraint. Comparing the two rows of Fig. 4.3, it can be seen that the two models achieve the same global optimum through different optimization paths: the SGDM curve changed topology twice, whereas the TGDM curve maintains the same topology throughout the entire evolution. It is important to notice that the TGDM curve is able to evolve out of an unfavorable configuration formed during the early stages, and that the topology constraint takes effect early but is released automatically later in the evolution. This demonstrates that the TGDM curve was not "jammed" by the topology constraint into the configuration of Fig. 4.3(h) or Fig. 4.3(i); instead, it successfully converges to the global optimum.

Fig. 4.4 shows another 2D example in which the SGDM and the TGDM geodesic active contour models used in previous experiment were applied again to find the boundary of a hand-shaped object. The original image (220×190 pixels) and the initial curve are shown in both Fig. 4.4(a) and Fig. 4.4(e). Figs. 4.4(b) and 4.4(c) show the SGDM contour at an intermediate and the final stage, respectively. Because the two middle fingers touch, the initial curve changes topology and splits into two separate curves as the final result (a larger outer curve and a disjoint inner curve as

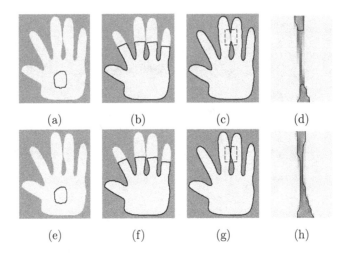

(a)   (b)   (c)   (d)

(e)   (f)   (g)   (h)

Figure 4.4: Segmentation of a hand phantom using both SGDM (top row) and TGDM (bottom row).

shown in Fig. 4.4(c) and zoomed up in Fig. 4.4(d)). We note that the two middle fingers in the hand become one "finger" with a hole in it in the final segmentation, which is obviously an undesirable result. The corresponding deformations of the TGDM contour are illustrated in Figs. 4.4(f) and 4.4(g). TGDM keeps the boundary of each finger separated, and the final contour correctly reflects the shape of the hand, as can be seen clearly in the zoomed view of Fig. 4.4(h).

As a final 2D example, we apply an SGDM model and the corresponding TGDM model to find the boundary of two adjacent bone cells in a CT image. The deformable model we adopt here is the binary-flow model proposed in [52]. The model applies a dynamic region force which tries to maximally separate the mean of the region encircled by the evolving contours from that of its complement. The curvature force is also used as a regularization force to counteract with the effect of image noise. Fig. 4.5(a) and 4.5(f) show the image overlaid with the initial curves. Without the topology constraint, the two separate curves merge at the weak gap between the two bone cells and one single contour that encloses both bones is produced as the final result. Again, the TGDM curves keep separated throughout the evolution and

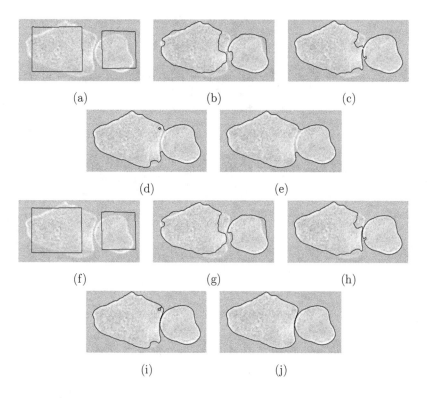

Figure 4.5: Segmentation of a carpal bones CT image using both SGDM and TGDM. (a) and (f): the initialization; (b)–(e): evolution of the SGDM contour; (g)–(j): evolution of the TGDM contour. (Original image courtesy of B. Kimia [1].)

correctly find the boundary of each cell.

4.4.2 3D experiments

In 3D, human brain mapping is a promising area to apply our new topology-preserving deformable model. More detailed discussion will be presented in the next chapter. In the following, we present the results from two 3D experiments for illustration purposes.

For the first 3D example, we applied a 3D version of the geometric deformable

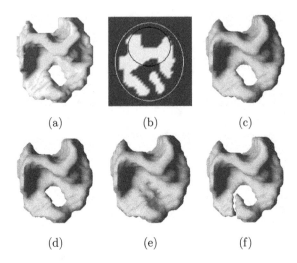

(a)   (b)   (c)

(d)   (e)   (f)

Figure 4.6: (a) A 3D phantom, (b) large sphere and small ellipsoid initializations, (c) SDGM result from sphere, (d) SGDM result from ellipsoid, (e) TGDM result from sphere, and (f) TGDM result from ellipsoid.

model of (2.11) to find the boundary surface of the 3D object depicted in Fig. 4.6(a). The object is actually a piece of a white matter segmented from an MR brain image. Due to data noise, the white matter piece has a handle, which is the wrong topology from an anatomical standpoint. In fact, we desire a topology equivalent to that of a sphere. We applied both SGDM and TGDM starting from two different initializations: a large sphere that encloses the whole object and a small ellipsoid that intersects with the object. A 2D slice showing the object and the two initial surfaces is shown in Fig. 4.6(b).

Figs. 4.6(c) and 4.6(d) are the final surfaces obtained by SGDM. The two results are the same since standard geometric deformable models are insensitive to initialization. The final surface has a handle, however, which is the incorrect topology. With the sphere as the initialization, TGDM gives the final surface shown in Fig. 4.6(e), and with the ellipsoid, it gives the result shown in Fig. 4.6(f). Both surfaces have the correct topology, but the topology is preserved in a different way. The surface obtained from the sphere initialization yields a thin membrane across the *tunnel* — a

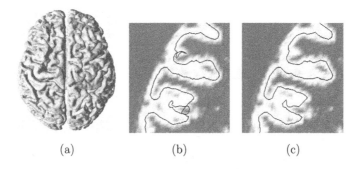

(a)   (b)   (c)

Figure 4.7: (a) Result of cortical surface reconstruction. (b) Self-intersection from PDM, and (c) no intersection with TGDM.

handle in the background image — through the original object, while the ellipsoid initialization makes a cut in the handle. The dependency of TGDM on its initialization is discussed in detail in the next section.

Our second 3D experiment applies SGDM, TGDM, and a parametric deformable surface model (PDM) to extract the central cortical surface from an initial fuzzy segmentation of a brain MR image volume. We used exactly the same initialization (a topologically correct surface near the gray-matter/white-matter interface), the same external forces, and similar internal forces for the geometric deformable models and the PDM. The results are presented in Fig. 4.7. Fig. 4.7(a) shows the final surface extracted from the parametric model. The SGDM and TGDM surfaces look identical at this level of detail, but on close examination there are important differences. The parametric model result, for example, has self-intersections, as shown in Fig. 4.7(b), while the TGDM surface does not, as shown in Fig. 4.7(c). Also, the SGDM result has 40 handles, whereas both the PDM and TGDM results have no handles and hence are topologically equivalent to spheres. Thus, TGDM produces both the correct topology and a valid manifold; hence it is the only model that gives a legal cortical surface reconstruction.

4.5 Discussion

Several issues are worthy of further investigation, which includes the dependency of the final segmentation results on different initializations, the computational complexity of imposing the topology constraint, and some related investigations in the literature.

The example shown in Fig. 4.6 points out a weakness in our overall approach that should be addressed in future work. First, the result can clearly depend on the initialization in a dramatic way. The two results, one that fills the tunnel and the other that breaks the handle, are dramatically different ways to address the issue of topology preservation. At present we have no formulation of an optimality criterion that would choose one of these solutions over the other. This situation is not atypical in deformable models, where the particular initialization very often determines the exact details of the final solution. As a step towards reducing the dependency on particular initialization, one can drop the topology constraint initially, that is, apply the standard geometric model to achieve an initial unconstrained optimal solution. After the unconstrained optimum is obtained, one can then apply a topology correction method to "project" the temporary solution back to the feasible domain, and start the constrained deformation from this "better" initialization. As one example, we applied the GTCA topology correction method on the SGDM result of Fig. 4.6(c) (which is also shown in Fig. 4.8(a) for clarity) to get the initialization shown in Fig. 4.8(b). The TGDM model then produced the final result as shown in Fig. 4.8(c). The new result is similar to that of Fig. 4.6(f), but it is now the unique solution, independent of initialization. This example actually illustrate the need of using GTCA to get a good initialization for the TGDM method, as is the approach we take in developing the cortical surface reconstruction procedure to be described in the next chapter. However, we note that such a topology correction (projection) method is not generally available for all topologies (the particular method can only be used to achieve a spherical topology), and when such an approach is taken, the initialization is determined by the optimality criterion applied in the topology correction method.

We note that the topological numbers are computed locally, which makes the

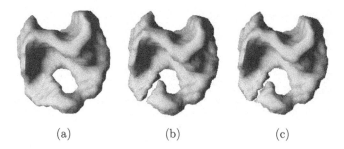

(a)   (b)   (c)

Figure 4.8: (a) The final result without topology constraint (SGDM), (b) initialization by topology correction, and (c) final result with TGDM.

simple point checking process straightforward and efficient. As a result, the topology constraint does not add much computational burden as compared to the standard narrow band implementation. For the phantom experiments, the time difference between standard and new geometric models are barely noticeable; and for the brain cortical surface reconstruction, the extra time taken by the topology constraint enforcement is less than 7 percent of the total processing time.

A related work is the shock detection method of [158, 159]. It is known from the Morse theory [160] that the implicit contour (zero level set of a level set function) undergoes topology changes if a critical point (extremal or saddle point) of the level set function, known as a *shock* point in [158, 159], passes through the zero level set, or in other words, it changes sign (see also [161]). Although the shock detection algorithm is promising in analyzing static shapes, it is time-consuming and unreliable in detecting and tracing sign changes of all shocks of a level set function evolving under a general velocity field, especially in 3D. One reason is that the level set function is sampled on discrete grids while its critical points are usually located between grid lines. In the topology-preserving mechanism proposed in this chapter, the topology change is directly correlated with sign-change of the level set function itself on the grid points, which provides a simple way to detect and prevent topology changes. However, the level set function itself is still evolving continuously, thus subpixel accuracy is maintained.

Another related work is the skeletally-coupled deformable model proposed by Sebastian et al. [1] for 2D carpal bone image segmentation. In this work, each bone cell is represented by a distinctly labeled region, and no two regions are allowed to merge during a seeded region growing. This approach only deals with one type of topological change — the merging of two disjoint regions. It cannot be easily generalized to deal with the splitting of a single region like the example shown in Fig. 4.4, nor can it be generalized to deal with one single region developing a handle in 3D. Overall, we believe that the most efficient and straightforward way to guarantee topology preservation in a deformable model algorithm is by applying the simple point criterion, as we have proposed herein.

4.6   Summary

In summary, we have developed a novel topology-preserving level set method and from which we derived a new class of geometric deformable models where the topology of the implicit curves or surfaces is preserved throughout the deformation. The topology is preserved by checking a simple point criterion during the level set evolution, which requires a relatively straightforward modification to the standard narrow band implementation of the traditional level set method. We have also shown that for energy minimizing geometric deformable models, their topology-preserving counterpart is a special constrained gradient descent algorithm that does not suffer from the jamming effect and is guaranteed to converge to a constrained optimal point of the energy functional. Several 2D and 3D experiments were conducted to show the success of the new models and illustrate their potential applications.

Chapter 5

Cortical Surfaces Reconstruction from MR Brain Images

In this chapter, we describe a systematic method to reconstruct the inner, the central, and the outer surfaces of the cerebral cortex from 3D MR brain images (cf. Fig. 1.4). Cortical surface reconstruction is a difficult task due to various imaging artifacts, and the complicated geometry of the cortex. To achieve a satisfactory reconstruction, the method must be both robust to imaging artifacts and able to capture the details of cortical geometry. Another important requirement is that the final surface representation have the correct topology and be a valid manifold without self-intersections.

In previous work, our group has developed a largely automatic multi-stage procedure for this task [2]. The method combines a fuzzy segmentation algorithm, an isosurface algorithm, and a parametric deformable surface model. The method described here is based on a similar design philosophy, but addresses some remaining limitations of the previous method, such as the deficiency in the previous median-filtering based topology correction approach, the requirement for manual editing to mask out subcortical structures, the existence of self-intersections in the final surface meshes, and the long computation time. The improvements are largely due to the application of the topology correction method and the topology preserving geometric deformable model introduced in the previous chapters. Two additional new components have also been developed: an automatic subcortical editing method which replaces the previous manual editing procedure and an anatomically consistent GM enhancement algorithm which overcomes the limitations of the partial volume effect. In addition, the new method reconstructs two additional cortical surfaces, the GM/WM surface and the GM/CSF (pial) surface. With these improvements, the current method is more accurate, faster and numerically more stable, and provides a complete characterization of the brain cortex. It is fully automatic except for some minimal manual interactions in the skull-stripping stage and for the manual picking of two anatomical landmark points, the anterior commissure (AC) and the posterior commissure (PC).

The chapter is organized as follows. We first survey in Section 5.1 the available cortical surface reconstruction methods in the literature, and make comparisons with our proposed method. We then describe our method in detail in Section 5.2. In Section 5.3, we present and discuss both the qualitative and quantitative results of applying our method to real MR brain data sets. Finally, we summarize the chapter in Section 5.4.

5.1 Related Work

Numerous approaches have been proposed in the literature for the reconstruction of cortex from MR brain images. These approaches differ in their ability to capture the convoluted cortical geometry, the reconstruction accuracy, the robustness against imaging artifacts, and whether they can produce a valid cortical representation that has the correct topology and has no self-intersections. For example, methods relying on tracing 2D contours through consecutive 2D image slices have difficulty in maintaining the consistency between slices, and in controlling the final surface topology. Thus, such methods are inadequate for the cortical reconstruction problem, although they can be helpful for generating truth models to evaluate the accuracy of other methods. Typical region-growing methods are limited in accuracy by the image voxel size. On the other hand, deformable surface models are able to deform through a continuum and yield a smooth surface representation of the cortex. However, standard parametric deformable models suffer from self-intersections, and traditional geometric deformable models lack topology control. In the following, we summarize representative works in this research area, and comment on the major weakness of each method if applicable. We focus on 3D algorithms, due to the clear drawback of 2D processing methods for this application.

The works by Mangin et al. [13] and Teo et al. [139] reconstruct the cortex using voxel-based approaches, and both methods pay special care to the topology correctness of the reconstruction results. The method by Mangin et al. [13] aims to construct a structural representation of the cortical topography, resulting in a relational network of major cortical sulci. The authors acknowledged the difficulty of finding the GM/CSF interface due to the partial volume effect. To address this issue, they segmented out the union of GM and CSF and then detected sulcal folds as the "excrescence" (outer skeleton) of the GM and CSF combination. They noted that the traditional deformable models had difficulty in capturing narrow cortical folds and could easily develop self-intersections. Thus, they proposed a method called the *homotopically deformable region growing* that combines a topologically constrained region growing with a Markov-random-field-like regularization scheme. As we explained in Section 3.1 of Chapter 3, this homotopically deformable region growing method has the effect of a topology correction algorithm, but the topological corrections it makes are arbitrarily located. As can be seen from the results presented in [13], their method led to unnatural long cuts inside the brain area. In our method, we apply a more carefully designed topology correction algorithm that optimally detects and removes topological defects; the same strategy has also been adopted by others [140, 162]. Another shortcoming of homotopic region growing is that its accuracy is limited to the voxel level and is therefore not well-suited for finding the pial surface.

Teo et al. [139] first segment out the WM and CSF structures using a maximum a posteriori (MAP) classifier with user-specified model parameters. After anisotropic diffusion and binarization, the resulting WM segmentation is manually checked for topological defects and corrected if they exist. Finally, a connected representation of the GM is created by a constrained region growing starting from the WM boundary.

Weaknesses of this method are that its accuracy is also limited to the voxel level, and the partial volume effect may cause many voxels to be misclassified. Furthermore, the amount of user interaction is very large, especially in the manual topology correction step.

The work by Davatzikos and Bryan [163] was among the first to apply 3D deformable surface model to the cortical surface reconstruction problem. This work directly models the brain cortex as a convoluted sheet of finite width, and applies a center-of-mass force to drive the surface to the geometric center of the cortical sheet. The force is computed from a binarized GM segmentation, and hence the accuracy is limited. A major drawback of this method lies in its inability to fully capture cortical folds, and thus an extra step is necessary to find the detailed sulcal structures [163, 164]. The results, however, no longer constitute a single coherent surface representation of the cortex.

Sandor and Leahy [116] developed a method to find and label the outer surface of the brain. Their method first extracts the brain using a combination of edge detection and morphological operations. Next, voxels corresponding to sulci are found in each 2D slice as sets of edge voxels forming cavities inside the brain surface but also connected to the surface. A deformable surface model is applied to register the extracted brain surface to an atlas model, and the anatomical labels are then transferred to the extracted surface. The brain surface found in this method, however, is only an approximate representation of the cortex, and does not correspond to any particular cortical surface.

Joshi et al. [165] developed a semiautomatic method to find the GM/WM interface. The work focused on macaque brain images, but the method was also tested on cryosectional image data from the Visible Human project. The method performs tissue segmentation by first fitting the image histogram with a mixture model, and then applying a maximum likelihood classifier using the estimated tissue parameters. To compensate for image intensity inhomogeneities, the histogram fitting and the classifier are computed locally in a neighborhood of each voxel. The WM boundary surface is then generated by an isosurface algorithm, and the surface topology is corrected by manual editing on the tissue segmentation. This editing step can take up to several days, as indicated in the paper.

The method developed by Dale et al. [28, 36] reconstructs both the inner and the outer cortical surfaces in a largely automatic manner. The method first corrects the intensity inhomogeneity of MR images by normalizing the WM peaks across 2D image slices. After removal of extracranial tissue by a deformable template model, the tissue segmentation is performed by intensity thresholding and post-filtering with oriented order-statistic filters. A surface tessellation of the segmented WM then produces an initial estimate of the GM/WM interface, which is refined using a parametric deformable surface model. The GM/WM surface is then deformed to find the GM/CSF interface. Self-intersection is explicitly checked and prevented during the surface deformations, but the final surface topology is corrected by manual editing. A weakness of this method is the simple intensity thresholding method that is used for the tissue segmentation. As can be seen in the presented results in [36], the subcortical GM structures tend to be misclassified as WM. The success of their method also relies on high image contrast; the data used in their experiments were obtained from averaging multiple scans of the same subject, thus placing extra requirement on the data acquisition step.

The difficulty in estimating the pial surface is explicitly handled in the approaches of Zeng et al. [34] and MacDonald et al. [35], by applying a tight thickness constraint within coupled surface propagation strategies. In both methods, the inner and the outer surfaces are reconstructed simultaneously, and the thickness constraint keeps the two surfaces at a close distance. As a result, the inner surface can help pull the outer surface inside narrow sulcal folds. On the other hand, inaccuracy in either surface can have an adverse effect on the accuracy of the other one. In addition, the assumption of a constant cortical thickness may bias the estimation of the true thickness [35, 166]. While the two methods both employ thickness constraints, they differ in the type of deformable surface models they adopt and the derivation of image forces for the surfaces deformation, as detailed next.

The method by Zeng et al. [34] applies a geometric deformable model, where each surface is embedded as the zero level set of a 3D signed distance function. In addition to the coupling between the two surfaces through the thickness constraint, each surface is driven by its own image-derived force towards the cortical boundary location. The boundary candidates are initially estimated by a local probabilistic model with pre-defined tissue intensity distributions. In order to employ this intensity distribution model, each image is first preprocessed to correct for intensity inhomogeneities and the resulting image histogram is normalized to have fixed peak intensity values. The method's main drawback is its lack of topology control in the geometric deformable surface model. Thus the reconstructed surfaces are not guaranteed to have the desired spherical topology. Some other methods based on similar techniques suffer from the same topology problem [167].

The method by MacDonald et al. [35] employs a coupled parametric deformable surface model, which does guarantee the topology correctness of the final surfaces. In addition to the thickness constraint that controls the relative distance of the two surfaces and prevents them from crossing each other, a self-proximity term is also added to prevent the occurrence of surface self-intersections. Drawbacks of this method include a possible bias caused by the global thickness constraint and very slow computation time due to the enforcement of self-intersection prevention (the method took about 30 hours). Also, the method does not separate the ventricles and subcortical structures from the cortex, and the reconstructed surfaces have many extraneous parts attached. This problem also exists in Zeng et al.'s results [34].

Kriegeskorte and Goebel [140] proposed using a similar approach as the method by Dale et al. [28, 36] to reconstruct the inner and the outer surfaces of the brain cortex, and they developed an automatic topology correction algorithm to replace the manual editing procedure of Dale et al. [28, 36]. The paper focuses mainly on the topology correction method, while the performance of the overall cortical surface reconstruction method was barely discussed.

Shattuck and Leahy [162] developed a system called BrainSuite for extracting the GM/WM interface from MR brain images. The multi-stage process first extracts the brain using the aforementioned Sandor and Leahy method [116]. After intensity inhomogeneity correction, the extracted brain volume is segmented into six classes that include both pure tissue classes and mixtures arising from the partial volume effect. Special care is taken to isolate the cortical WM and fill the inside cavities corresponding to the ventricles and subcortical GM structures, which involves some necessary manual editing. Topology correction is then performed on the binarized version of the edited WM volume, and finally an isosurface algorithm is applied to get the WM boundary surface with the correct topology. The method does not try to estimate the pial surface due to the acknowledged difficulty in identifying the sulcal banks within tight sulci.

Xu et al. [2] proposed a largely automatic procedure for reconstructing the central layer of the human cerebral cortex. After preprocessing the data to extract the cerebrum, the brain image is segmented into membership functions of GM, WM, and CSF tissue classes using an adaptive fuzzy C-means algorithm that simultaneously estimates an intensity inhomogeneity field. After manually filling in the cavities of WM corresponding to ventricles and subcortical GM structures, iterated median filtering of the WM membership volume is performed until its boundary surface has the correct spherical topology. This initial estimate of the cortical surface is then deformed towards the central layer of the cortex using a parametric deformable model, which preserves the topology of the initial surface. The method has several disadvantages. First, the tissue classification algorithm used, although robust to intensity inhomogeneity, can be sensitive to image noise. Second, the median filtering approach for topology correction tends to oversmooth the initial surface and is not guaranteed to converge. Third, the method has difficulty in capturing narrow sulci due to the partial volume effect. Finally, although the deformable model preserves surface topology, it may produce self-intersections. As introduced previously, in this work we improve upon the previous method by addressing all these disadvantages.

5.2 Methods

In this section, we present our new method for reconstructing the GM/WM interface, the central cortical surface, and the pial surface (GM/CSF interface) from T1-weighted MR images of the brain. The overall principle is similar to some existing methods, which combine low-level tissue classification and deformable surface model based surface reconstruction. However, there are important differences in the details,

114

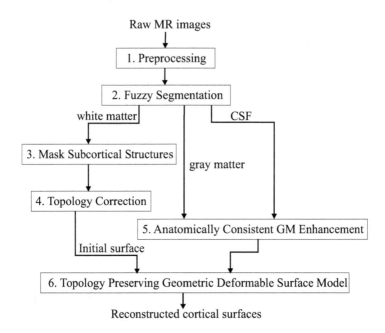

Figure 5.1: Block diagram of the overall cortical surface reconstruction system.

which will become clear in the following. A block diagram of the overall method is shown in Fig. 5.1. The procedure begins with an MR image data set that undergoes a preprocessing step to isolate the brain volume by removing extracranial tissue. This is followed by a tissue classification step that segments the remaining image regions into GM, WM, and CSF. A mask is automatically generated to fill in the cavities inside the WM corresponding to ventricles and subcortical GM structures. The resulting WM volume is processed by the GTCA topology correction algorithm to make sure its boundary surface has the desired spherical topology; this produces the initial estimate of the GM/WM interface. This surface is further deformed to find the three cortical surfaces in sequence using the TGDM method. To allow the central and the pial surfaces better capture narrow cortical folds, an anatomically consistent enhancement of GM is used to force evidence of CSF where it otherwise might not appear due to partial volume averaging. We now describe each of these steps in sequence.

5.2.1 Data acquisition and preprocessing

Our procedure uses T1-weighted volumetric MR brain images with voxel size $0.9375 \times 0.9375 \times 1.5$mm. This data provides adequate contrast between GM, WM, and CSF in a single intensity parameter, and has fine enough resolution to resolve the complex structure of the cortex.

After the image data has been acquired, it is preprocessed to remove skin, bone, fat, and other non-cerebral tissue using a semi-automated software package developed by Christos Davatzikos and Jerry Miller at Johns Hopkins University [168]. This package features a combination of region growing algorithms and mathematical morphology operators to ease the processing of cerebral tissue extraction. Next, the cerebellum and brain stem are removed since we are only interested in the cerebral cortex. Currently, this is performed manually but we note that further automation in these steps may be possible using other published methods [4,162,169]. Fig. 5.2 shows two slices from a typical MR image volume before and after this procedure was applied. The increased contrast apparent in the last two images is simply the result

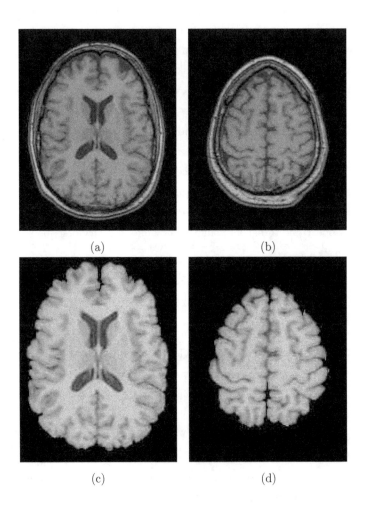

(a)　　　　　　　　　　(b)

(c)　　　　　　　　　　(d)

Figure 5.2: Sample slices from acquired MR image data and preprocessed data: (a)-(b) two slices from original MR acquisition, (c)-(d) same slices after preprocessing to extract cerebrum.

of an image intensity rescaling. The final step in the preprocessing is to trilinearly interpolate the stripped brain volume to cubic voxels having the in-plane resolution in all three directions. This reduces the directional dependency in subsequent processing stages.

5.2.2 Tissue classification

Once the MR images have been preprocessed, a tissue classification algorithm is employed to identify the image regions corresponding to GM, WM, and CSF. The algorithm we used is called the Fuzzy and Noise Tolerant Adaptive Segmentation Method (FANTASM), which was developed and programmed by Dzung Pham [170]. FANTASM is an improved version of the Adaptive Fuzzy C-Means (AFCM) algorithm used in the previous central cortical surface reconstruction method [2]. Like AFCM, FANTASM generates a fuzzy segmentation while compensating for intensity inhomogeneity artifacts that may occur within the MR images. The advantage of FANTASM over AFCM is the increased robustness against image noise due to the incorporation of a spatial smoothness constraint on the resulting membership functions.

The output of FANTASM is illustrated in Fig. 5.3; it produces three fuzzy membership functions for the three tissue classes. We note that the membership functions are continuous-valued functions with values in the range of $[0, 1]$, which reflect the degree of similarity between the observed intensity at every image voxel and the mean intensities (called *centroids*) of the three tissue classes. In addition, the three membership functions add up to one at every image voxel location, and thus provide an indication of fractional tissue contributions for each voxel. For example, at a homogeneous voxel that contains only one tissue type, the membership function of the corresponding tissue class will have a value equal to one, and the other two membership values will both be zero. A voxel that has more than one non-zero membership values contains a mixture of different tissue classes, which indicates that it is located near a boundary between multiple tissue types. Assuming that every voxel can contain at most two tissue types, which is generally true around the brain cortex, we can estimate the tissue boundaries as the voxel locations where two of the

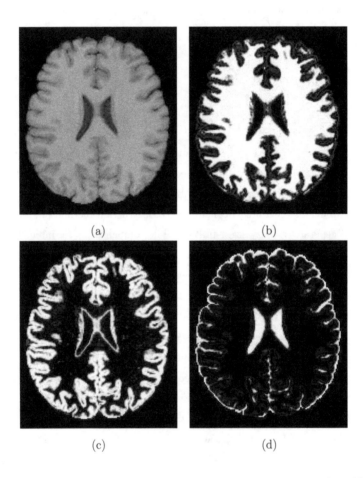

(a)

(b)

(c)

(d)

Figure 5.3: 2D slice view of the tissue classification results using FANTASM: (a) original brain image after preprocessing, (b) WM membership, (c) GM membership, and (d) CSF membership.

three membership functions are non-zero and both equal to 0.5 (since they sum up to one). Typically, such an estimation can be achieved by an interpolation procedure, either explicitly as in an isosurface algorithm, or implicitly through the image force applied in a deformable model based boundary segmentation method. Both types of approaches are utilized in our cortical surface reconstruction method.

As demonstrated in [170], FANTASM provides very accurate tissue segmentation results; however, as with other low level image segmentation methods, it does not directly produce a coherent and consistent estimation of the cortical surfaces. Although a simple surface tessellation of the WM membership function by an isosurface algorithm can give a quite accurate estimation of the GM/WM interface, such a surface usually does not have the correct topology, often having a large number of handles. Also, some extraneous surfaces from the subcortical structures will be wrongly attached to this WM isosurface. In addition, correctly estimating the central and the pial surfaces is still problematic within sulcal regions due to the partial volume effect. As can be seen from the GM segmentation result, the partial volume effect still causes adjacent GM banks within a narrow sulcus to be hardly distinguishable. These issues will be addressed in the following steps. We note that all later steps use the fuzzy membership functions as a concrete representation of the original image, with the image noise and intensity inhomogeneity artifacts already removed or largely reduced.

5.2.3 Automatic editing of the WM membership function

In this step of the algorithm, we aim to artificially close the hole at the bottom of the brain, in order to prevent the boundaries of the ventricles and the subcortical GM structures such as the putamen and the caudate nucleus from being connected to the estimated cortical surfaces. Since these structures all lie inside the WM, it is necessary to edit the initial WM segmentation to fill in the cavities corresponding to these structures (cf. Fig. 5.4). Such an editing was performed manually in the method reported by Xu et al. [2] and Shattuck et al. [162]. Manually editing is quite tedious. In this work, we proposed an automatic method, called AutoFill, to accomplish this

120

task, thereby reducing manual interaction and making the algorithm applicable to large population studies.

The main observation that serves as the basis of this method is that the subcortical GM together with the ventricles form cavities inside the WM that open towards the bottom of the brain. As illustrated in Fig. 5.4(c), such cavities that must be filled can be identified by the presence of the ventricles. To make use of this anatomical information, the ventricles are first extracted using a simple 3D geometric deformable surface model, which applies a regional signed pressure force and a smoothing curvature force. The signed pressure force is derived from the CSF membership function, which expands the surface at places where the membership value is larger than 0.5 and contracts if less than 0.5. The smoothing force prevents the surface from growing into the CSF outside the brain cortex (cf. Fig. 5.4(d)). The deformable model is initialized by a simple sphere centered at the centroid of the CSF membership volume. Although better initialization may be possible, we have found that the result is quite insensitive to the initial surface, and the ventricles need not be accurately segmented for the AutoFill purpose. An example of the segmented ventricle structure is shown in Fig. 5.5.

The next step of AutoFill uses the segmented ventricles as seeds, and applies a seeded region growing method to detect and fill the cavities inside a binarized WM volume. If directly performed in 3D, a region growing method would require an additional sealing plane to properly stop growing at the bottom of the brain. In general, it is hard to find such a sealing plane in the 3D volume due to the irregular shape of the brain. Instead, we found it possible to apply this same principle on 2D coronal slices, separately, and then merge these results into a 3D result. In this case, a horizontal "sealing line" is defined at the base of the brain within each coronal slice to stop the 2D seeded region growing method. The remaining task is to define how to properly select a sealing line in each coronal slice.

We found that there are in general three types of coronal slices to be dealt with. At the most anterior or posterior parts of the brain, the coronal slices do not go through the brain stem area, and the subcortical structures form perfect cavities in each coronal slice, and no additional sealing lines are needed. At the central parts of

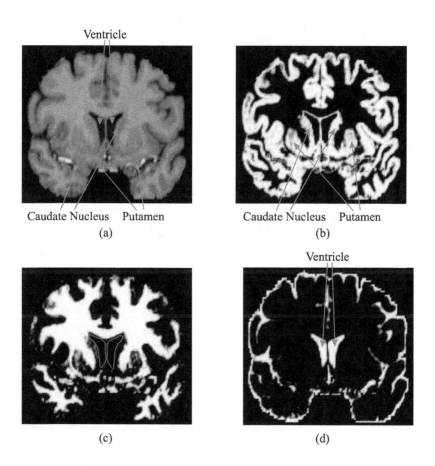

Figure 5.4: Illustration of subcortical structures on a coronal slice and its tissue segmentations. (a) is the original image; (b), (c), and (d) are the GM, WM, and CSF membership functions, respectively. The blue curves in (c) indicate the boundary of the ventricles.

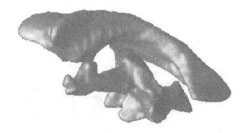

Figure 5.5: Surface rendering of the detected ventricles.

the brain, one additional sealing line suffices (although we will later discuss the need for a putamen mask in some cases to handle the possible leakage at the cortex next to the putamen region). The third type of coronal slices correspond to some posterior slices where the WM are separated into two hemispheres, and the region-growing must be performed in each hemisphere individually. We have designed a three-pass procedure to automatically handle all three cases. The details are described in the following:

First Pass. The first pass is the simplest. In each 2D coronal slice, region growing is used to find all background holes, and to fill them with WM if they contain part of the detected ventricles. Background holes are defined to be connected components of background voxels that are not adjacent to the image boundary. This pass typically fills subcortical regions in the anterior slices that do not pass through the brain stem. Some posterior slices are also filled if the ventricle regions form closed holes inside the WM. Fig. 5.6 shows one coronal slice that is correctly edited after the first pass.

The coronal slices in the center of the brain are not changed after the first pass because in this range the ventricles and subcortical GM are topologically connected to the slice boundary through the opening around the brain stem area, and thus the region growing in the first pass is unable to find a closed background region containing the detected ventricles. For these slices, a horizontal sealing line must be defined for each slice to provide a lower boundary for region growing. This is the task of the

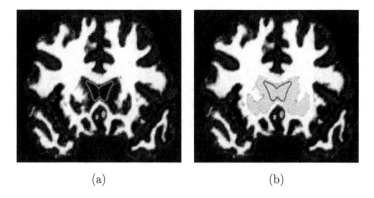

(a)   (b)

Figure 5.6: A coronal slice that gets correctly filled during the first pass. The blue curves show the detected ventricle boundary.

second pass.

Second Pass. The second pass starts by examining each coronal slice to see whether unfilled regions of ventricles exist. The existence of unfilled ventricles indicates that the subcortical regions are connected to the background outside and thus were not filled in the first pass. For each of these slices that remain to be filled, the algorithm selects a horizontal sealing line to help separating the subcortical regions from the rest of the background. One reasonable choice is to make the lines be aligned with the bottom of the diencephalon. Again, we could select a single sealing plane in the Talairach coordinate system and map it to the subject brain, which automatically defines a sealing line for each slice. In the current implementation, however, we adopt a more data-driven approach in which the sealing boundary is determined separately for each slice and is aligned with the "bottom" of the GM along the mid-sagittal line in the current slice.[9] More specifically, we search along the mid-sagittal line in the current slice from the bottom to the top until the first GM voxel is encountered. The horizontal sealing line is then defined to be passing through this point. Since the cerebellum and the brain stem were removed during the initial preprocessing step,

---

[9]The mid-sagittal line is the intersection of the coronal slice and the mid-sagittal plane — the sagittal plane that passes through the AC-PC line.

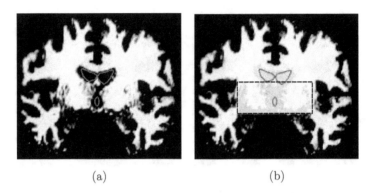

(a)   (b)

Figure 5.7: (a) The original WM slice and (b) the edited result (WM filled). The blue curves show the detected ventricle boundary and the dashed rectangular box shows the boundary of the putamen mask.

the line found this way is roughly aligned to the bottom of the diencephalon.

During the second pass, we address a difficulty that may arise when a thin strand of WM that exists between the putamen and the cortical GM is broken due to an error in tissue classification. This condition causes the region-growing procedure to fail, i.e., the region will grow onto the image boundary. The problem is addressed by applying a mask to identify the putamen region and constraining the region growing to take place within this mask. The mask is drawn *a priori* in Talairach coordinates [14] and is mapped automatically to each individual brain after the brain is registered to the standardized space using the method described in [171]. To initialize the registration, two landmark points are required: the anterior commissure (AC) and the posterior commissure (PC). Currently, the two landmark points are picked manually for each brain, which takes only a few minutes of operator time. We use the simple Talairach registration to define the putamen mask because the Talairach registration is known to be reliable in broad localization of subcortical structures. We apply the putamen mask when the seeded region growing with the additional sealing line fails to find a closed region for the slices within the range of the putamen mask. A central coronal slice that is edited with the help of the putamen mask is shown in Fig. 5.7.

Third Pass. The first two passes correctly fill most of the coronal slices except some posterior ones that are behind the PC, where the segmented WM separates into two disjoint hemispheres and thus the subcortical region is still connected to the background outside even with the additional sealing line. In these slices, we have to address the two hemispheres separately, which is the task of the third pass.

In these posterior slices, the regions that need to be filled correspond to the posterior horns of the lateral ventricle. These ventricular regions might already be correctly filled during the first pass if they form closed holes inside the WM, e.g., the ventricle hole on the left-hand side in Fig. 5.8(b). One extra issue arises due to the presence of a CSF structure known as the superior cistern in these slices. The superior cistern is typically included in the segmented ventricles, whose boundary corresponds to the middle blue curve in Figs. 5.8(a) and 5.8(b). This CSF structure does not need to be filled as WM. Thus, in order to correctly determine whether there are still ventricle regions that need to be filled, we first need to separate the superior cistern from the true ventricle horns in these slices.

One feature that can differentiate the ventricle horns from the superior cistern is location: the superior cistern lies around the mid-sagittal plane, while the ventricle horns lie separately in the two hemispheres. We extract the superior cistern in these slices by picking a ventricle-labeled point in the mid-sagittal line as a seed and then region-grow from it (in 2D) until all the ventricle-labeled voxels connected to it are relabeled as non-ventricle. The remaining ventricle-labeled voxels are considered to belong to the true ventricle horns. After separating the superior cistern from the true ventricle, we search for unfilled ventricle horns in the left and right hemisphere separately. If unfilled regions exist, they become the seeds for the third-pass region growing.

To fill the ventricle horn in either hemisphere, two sealing lines are usually required, one horizontal and one vertical. The position of the horizontal line is determined in the following way. First, draw a vertical line through each voxel that is labeled as ventricle. Then search along each line towards the bottom of the brain until a WM voxel is encountered. Next, among all the WM voxels found in the second step, take the one with the lowest vertical coordinate and draw a horizontal line passing

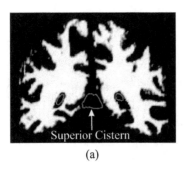 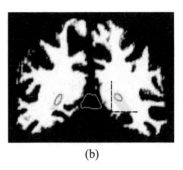

(a)   (b)

Figure 5.8: One posterior slice of the segmented WM volume (a) and its corresponding edited result (b). The dashed lines show the location of the sealing lines found for the right hemisphere.

through this point. The position of the vertical line is taken to be aligned with the rightmost (leftmost) boundary of the ventricle horn in the left (right) hemisphere. We then shift the vertical lines towards the mid-sagittal plane by 3 pixels in order to fill a bit more around the ventricle horns.

With the two sealing lines as additional boundaries, the region growing can successfully fill the regions occupied by the posterior ventricle horns. Fig. 5.8 shows one posterior coronal slice and the corresponding edited result.

The three pass procedure works well in practice. Figure 5.9 shows a typical example of the GM/WM interface obtained with and without the AutoFill procedure. AutoFill successfully closes the hole at the bottom of the brain, and the boundaries of the subcortical structures are no longer connected to the cortical surface. In addition, we have observed in our experiments that edited WM volumes often result in fewer topological inconsistencies that would otherwise have been present from inclusion of the putamen area.

5.2.4 Topology correction of WM isosurface

After AutoFill, a reasonable estimate of the GM/WM interface can be found by computing an isosurface of the edited WM membership function at the isovalue

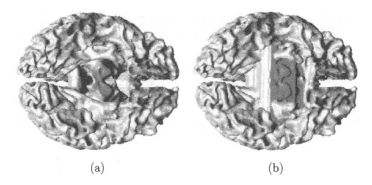

(a)   (b)

Figure 5.9: The GM/WM interfaces obtained from the original (a) and the edited (b) WM segmentation.

of 0.5. Unfortunately, this surface does not, in general, have the correct topology because of the presence of noise and partial volume averaging in the original MR image. Thus, in this step, we employ the GTCA algorithm that was developed in Chapter 3 to obtain a topologically correct WM boundary surface. This surface will serve as the initialization for the next topology-preserving surface deformation step to reconstruct the three cortical surfaces. Although the topology-preserving deformable surface model could be directly applied to get topologically correct surface reconstructions starting from a simpler initialization, e.g., a sphere, the topological barriers thus resulted in the final surfaces would be arbitrary and far from optimal, since the deformable model has little control over the locations where the handles are prevented from forming. Initialization problems are also found in other methods such as the homotopic region growing and parametric deformable model methods. Thus GTCA is used to generate a proper initialization for the deformable surface model, i.e., one that is very close to the desired surfaces. As demonstrated in Chapter 3, the GTCA algorithm locally and efficiently removes all the handles from an initial WM segmentation, and produces a topologically correct WM boundary surface identical to the original one except for small cuts or fills at the removed handle locations.

5.2.5 Anatomically consistent GM enhancement

The cortical folds of the GM/WM interface are more open than that of the other two surfaces. Thus, the inner cortical surface is relatively unaffected by the partial volume effect, and the topology-corrected isosurface can produce a very accurate representation of the inner cortical surface. Although estimation of the GM/WM interface is fairly straightforward, estimation of the GM/CSF interface and also the central surface is still problematic. Even on very high resolution scans, there are regions within sulci where the cortical gray matter is literally "back-to-back" — i.e., there is no evidence of separate sulcal GM banks at all. Without use of anatomical prior knowledge in these areas, estimating surface position, thickness, and other geometric measures related to the cortex would be widely inaccurate. This difficulty has also been recognized by other groups, as discussed in Section 5.1.

One way to address this problem is to impose a thickness constraint, which will not allow the cortical thickness to be larger than a certain threshold [34, 35]. There is evidence, however that this type of constraint may bias the true calculation of thickness [35, 166]. Another approach is to seek subtle evidence of CSF within the MR images and to accentuate the CSF signature within the folds [32]. When there truly is no evidence of CSF, however, this method will fail.

In this work, we propose an alternative approach, which we call the *anatomically consistent enhancement* (ACE). As illustrated in Fig. 5.10, the idea is to provide a GM representation that has evidence of sulci where the MR scanner might otherwise not reveal them. ACE is based on the anatomical knowledge that the GM is folded along the boundary of the WM, and within each sulcal fold, two GM banks should exist that are separated by CSF (cf. Fig. 5.10(a)). Thus, at a tight sulcus when the evidence of CSF is missing due to the partial volume effect and limited image resolution, ACE will modify the initial GM segmentation to create a thin (artificial) separation (cf. Fig. 5.10(b)–(c)).

As described in a preliminary report [172], ACE works by automatically locating the exterior skeleton of the GM/WM interface through a Euclidean distance transform, and reducing the GM membership function value at the skeletal points and

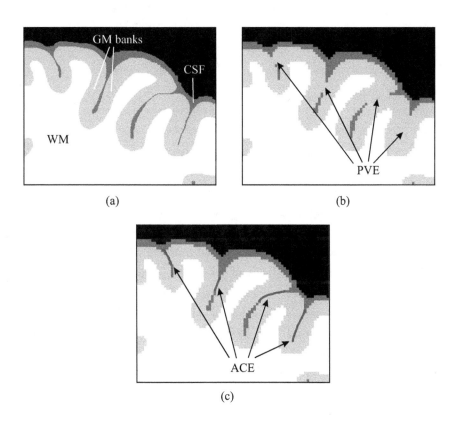

Figure 5.10: Illustration of the partial volume effect (PVE) and ACE. (a) Ideal image showing the correct cortical geometry. (b) Sampled image with smeared sulcal folds. (c) "Gauging" by ACE to reveal separate sulcal banks.

changing it into CSF. A similar skeleton idea has been applied in [13] to directly define sulci from the union of GM and CSF. However, in ACE, the change in the membership functions only affects the estimation of the pial and the central surface indirectly. For example, if the skeletal points are already labeled as CSF, which is highly likely in a wide sulcus, the modification done by ACE will not have any effect at all. Also, unlike the global thickness constraint, the effect of ACE is automatically localized to sulcal regions, and does not affect the thickness computation at gyral regions.

Modifying the GM membership function at the outside Euclidean skeletal points of the WM membership is correct only if the GM banks are symmetric. If the initial segmentation shows only a solid GM block at a sulcus with no evidence of CSF at all, then this simple change is the best choice we can make. In general, however, the symmetric assumption is not true, as might be indicated by some evidence of CSF within a sulcus. In such cases, the simple change can lead to a "gouging" that is not in the correct position, as predicted by the CSF information. This is illustrated in Fig. 5.11(a). In such cases, we would like the skeletal points to reside inside the CSF. This can be accomplished by using a weighted distance function to define the skeletal or equal-distance points; that is, distance across CSF area will be assigned larger values than the true Euclidean distance. For example, in Fig. 5.11(b), such a weighted distance measure will essentially imply that $a = b$ and $c = d$. In regions where there is no evidence of CSF, the distance will default back to the Euclidean one. We now describe how to implement such a weighted distance transform.

In general, a weighted distance function can be computed by solving the following Eikonal equation:

$$
\begin{aligned}
F(\mathbf{x})|\nabla D(\mathbf{x})| &= 1 \text{ in } \Omega, \\
D(\mathbf{x}) &= 0 \text{ for } \mathbf{x} \in \Gamma,
\end{aligned}
\tag{5.1}
$$

where $F(\mathbf{x})$ is a spatially varying speed function defined within the computational domain Ω, and Γ is the surface from which the weighted distance $D(\mathbf{x})$ is measured. If the speed function $F(\mathbf{x})$ is unity at every point, then $D(\mathbf{x})$ reduces to the Euclidean distance measure. This Eikonal equation can be solved efficiently using an $O(N \log N)$ algorithm known as the *fast marching method* (FMM) [55, 121].

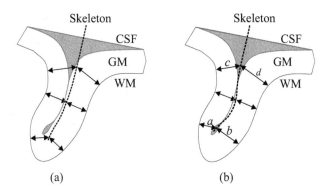

Figure 5.11: (a) The true skeleton under Euclidean distance measure. (b) The preferred skeleton location for ACE.

For the computation of ACE, Γ corresponds to the GM/WM interface. Since topology correctness is not important when computing ACE, we take as Γ the 0.5-isosurface of the WM membership function (after AutoFill has been run), slightly smoothed using a geometric curvature flow [55]. To compute the CSF-weighted distance function D_{csf}, we define the speed function $F(\mathbf{x})$ as a function of the CSF membership function:

$$F(\mathbf{x}) = 1 - 0.9\mu_{\mathrm{csf}}(\mathbf{x}), \tag{5.2}$$

where $\mu_{\mathrm{csf}}(\mathbf{x})$ denotes the CSF fuzzy membership function (whose value falls in the range of $[0, 1]$). Thus, over CSF areas, the speed is low, and the distance increment is larger than the Euclidean distance measure.

The skeletal points of D_{csf} are then computed. Let $S(\mathbf{x}) = F(\mathbf{x})|\nabla D_{\mathrm{csf}}(\mathbf{x})|$. The skeletal points are where the equality $S(\mathbf{x}) = 1$ does not hold; instead, $S(\mathbf{x}) \ll 1$ at these points. Thus, we can locate the skeletal points by comparing $S(\mathbf{x})$ against the value one. In order to be robust to numerical errors, we typically use the threshold 0.8 instead of unity.

The effect of using a weighted distance transform for the skeleton computation is illustrated in Fig. 5.12 with a 2D phantom. The white U-shaped object in Fig. 5.12(a) represents a sulcus, and the small gray object lies in-between represents the CSF

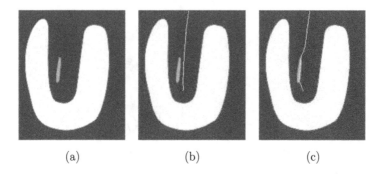

(a)   (b)   (c)

Figure 5.12: (a) A 2D sulcus phantom. (b) The exterior skeleton of the U-shape computed using the Euclidean distance measure. (c) The exterior skeleton computed when using the weighted distance measure.

evidence. Fig. 5.12(b) shows in yellow the exterior skeleton of the U-shaped object when using the Euclidean distance measure. The skeleton computed using the CSF-weighted distance function is shown in yellow in Fig. 5.12(c); it is clear that the skeleton is shifted to follow the evidence of CSF within the region.

To create the anatomy consistent separation of sulcal banks, we modify the initial GM membership function using the function $S(\mathbf{x})$. In particular, we define

$$\mu'_{\mathrm{GM}}(\mathbf{x}) = \begin{cases} S(\mathbf{x})\mu_{\mathrm{GM}}(\mathbf{x}) & S(\mathbf{x}) < 0.8 \\ \mu_{\mathrm{GM}}(\mathbf{x}) & \text{otherwise,} \end{cases} \tag{5.3}$$

where μ_{GM} and μ'_{GM} denote the initial and enhanced GM membership functions, respectively. The 0.8 threshold is applied to eliminate noise caused by numerical errors. Note that we only perform the above modification outside of the GM/WM interface, i.e., at exterior skeletal points of the GM/WM interface.

A cross-sectional view of a 3D ACE result is shown in Fig. 5.13. Clearly, there is a marked improvement in the appearance of sulcal gaps in the ACE result as compared to the original GM membership function. We note that ACE does not make any assumptions about the maximum cortical thickness, so it will not restrict the cortical width anywhere in the cortex. We also note that it only has an effect within sulci, and even then only when there is actual gray matter on the outside skeleton. Overall,

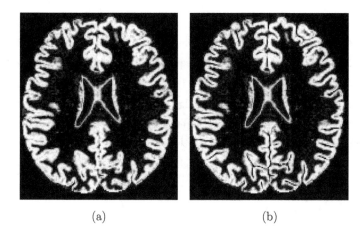

(a)   (b)

Figure 5.13: (a) Original GM membership function and (b) the ACE enhanced GM membership function.

we consider ACE to be a better solution to the partial volume problem than using a thickness constraint.

5.2.6   Nested surface reconstruction using TGDM

After the topology correction of the WM isosurface using GTCA and the enhancement of the membership function using ACE, we are now ready to extract all three cortical surfaces. We achieve this by applying a deformable surface model. It is imperative that the deformable model maintain the topology of the surface and not creating surface abnormalities such as self-intersections. The topology correctness could be accomplished using parametric deformable surface models, but the detection and prevention of self-intersections would be difficult and time-consuming. In Chapter 4, we described TGDM, a new class of topology-preserving geometric deformable models, and showed that it inherits the advantages of traditional geometric deformable models with the added property of maintaining the model topology. In particular, like traditional geometric deformable models, the contour deformation in TGDM is computed implicitly, and the self-intersection problem is automatically

134

circumvented.

In the current application, three implementations of TGDM are utilized to extract the inner, central, and pial surfaces in sequence. TGDM for the inner surface aims to improve the surface accuracy around the topological corrections and to slightly regularize the isosurface, which can be noisy due to imaging artifacts. When extracting the central and pial surfaces, an additional constraint is added to the TGDM implementation to ensure the proper nesting of the surfaces. We now describe how to design the model parameters and image forces that will drive the surface models to their desired surface locations.

5.2.7 Refinement of the GM/WM surface

The first TGDM model is targeted at refining the GM/WM surface. To accomplish this, we use TGDM with a curvature force and a regional signed pressure force; the advection force $F_{\text{adv}}(\mathbf{x})$ in (2.10) is not needed. The curvature force aims to regularize the surface, and is proportional to the mean curvature $\kappa(x)$ of the surface. The signed pressure force is defined as

$$R(x) = 2\mu'_{\text{WM}}(x) - 1,$$

where μ'_{WM} denotes the new WM membership function after AutoFill. Since $\mu'_{\text{WM}} \in [0, 1]$, $R(x)$ falls in the range of $[-1, 1]$. If $\mu'_{\text{WM}} > 0.5$ then $R(x) > 0$, whereas if $\mu'_{\text{WM}} < 0.5$ then $R(x) < 0$. Therefore, $R(x)$ provides outward balloon forces when the surface resides within the WM and inward forces when it resides outside the WM. Thus, $R(x)$ will force the surface to the GM/WM boundary. The weights for the two forces are chosen to be $\omega_R = 1$ and $\omega_\kappa = -0.02$, determined empirically at present.

The initial surface is defined by the signed distance function computed from the 0.5-isosurface of the topology corrected WM volume. After convergence, the final level set function, denoted by Φ_{in}, is also a signed distance function, which embeds the final inner surface as its zero level set. An explicit tessellation of the final GM/WM interface is extracted by applying the CCMC algorithm with Φ_{in} as the input, as described in Chapter 4. TGDM guarantees that this surface has a spherical topology, which can be verified by checking the Euler number of the surface mesh.

5.2.8   Central cortical surface

The second TGDM model is designed to find the central cortical surface. As demonstrated in the work by Xu et al. [2], the use of a gradient vector flow (GVF) force makes it easy to find the central layer of a thick sheet. Suppose we take the GM membership function μ_{GM} itself as an edge map, and compute the gradient vector flow from it. Then, the resulting GVF force will point to the center of the thick "edge", that is, the center of the GM sheet. We use the ACE enhanced GM membership function μ'_{GM} to compute the GVF force in this work, which improves the accuracy of the central surface estimation and reduces the error caused by the partial volume effect around tight sulcal regions. Specifically, the GVF external force $\vec{v}(\mathbf{x})$ applied in this TGDM model is computed as the equilibrium solution of the following system of partial differential equations

$$\vec{v}_t(\mathbf{x}, t) = c\nabla^2 \vec{v}(\mathbf{x}, t) - (\vec{v}(\mathbf{x}, t) - \nabla\mu'_{\mathrm{GM}}(\mathbf{x}))|\nabla\mu'_{\mathrm{GM}}(\mathbf{x})|^2 , \qquad (5.4)$$

where $\vec{v}_t$ denotes the partial derivative of $\vec{v}(\mathbf{x}; t)$ with respect to t, ∇^2 is the Laplacian operator, and c is a weight, which we set to 0.2.

To make sure the surface does not move out of the cortex, we also apply a regional force similar to the one used in [2],

$$R_{\mathrm{cent}}(\mathbf{x}) = \begin{cases} 0, & \text{if } |2\mu'_{\mathrm{WM}}(\mathbf{x}) + \mu'_{\mathrm{GM}}(\mathbf{x}) - 1| < 0.5; \\ 2\mu'_{\mathrm{WM}}(\mathbf{x}) + \mu'_{\mathrm{GM}}(\mathbf{x}) - 1, & \text{otherwise.} \end{cases} \qquad (5.5)$$

This region force pushes the surface outward if it is in the WM, inward if in the CSF, but has no effect within the GM. Thus, the surface moves toward the central axis of the GM under the influence of GVF forces alone. We also apply a small curvature force to keep the surface smooth. The relative strengths of the individual forces are determined by their coefficients, which we fix to be $\omega_R = \omega_{\vec{v}} = 1$ and $\omega_\kappa = -0.02$ for all brain studies.

Using these internal and external forces, the central surface TGDM is applied starting from the previous TGDM output, Φ_{in}, which is the signed distance function from the GM/WM surface. A barrier constraint is implemented to prevent the central surface from moving inside the GM/WM interface, which might otherwise happen due to noise or numerical rounding errors. Under the convention of the signed distance function, it is easy to check that if the inner surface is to stay inside the central surface, then at every grid point the signed distance function for the central surface should have smaller value than that of the inner surface. Thus, during the narrow band update of the level set function Φ_{cent} for the central surface, we prevent its value from getting smaller than the initialization. In particular, we add an additional step immediately after Step 3(a) in Algorithm 4.1, in which we set $\Phi_{\text{temp}}(\mathbf{y}_i)$ to $\Phi_{\text{in}}(\mathbf{y}_i) + \epsilon$ if initially $\Phi_{\text{temp}}(\mathbf{y}_i) \leq \Phi_{\text{in}}(\mathbf{y}_i)$, where ϵ is a small positive number. This constraint keeps the central surface outside of the inner surface, and prevents the two surfaces from ever crossing.

5.2.9 Pial surface

The third and final TGDM is designed to find the pial surface starting from the central surface obtained in the last step. Based on the membership functions, the pial surface can be defined as the outer 0.5-isosurface of the cortical GM membership function. Since the cortical GM is sandwiched between WM and CSF, and totally surrounds the WM, the pial surface can also be defined as the 0.5-isosurface of the union of GM and WM. This second definition automatically distinguishes the pial surface from the GM/WM interface, which is the inner 0.5-isosurface of the cortical GM. Note that we need to use the WM membership function after AutoFill in the above definition, which will prevent the boundary of the ventricles from being wrongly connected to the pial surface. Also, we need to use the GM membership function after ACE to get a pial surface that captures deep sulcal folds.

We choose the image force for the pial surface TGDM as a signed pressure force, which is defined as follows:

$$R_{\text{out}}(\mathbf{x}) = 1 - 2(\mu'_{\text{GM}}(\mathbf{x}) + \mu'_{\text{WM}}(\mathbf{x})),$$

where μ'_{WM} is the WM membership function after AutoFill, and μ'_{GM} is the ACE-modified GM membership function. This region force makes the surface expand if it is in the WM or GM and contract if it is in the CSF. Mean curvature is still used as the internal force, and no advection force is used in this TGDM. The weights are chosen as before to be $\omega_R = 1$ and $\omega_\kappa = -0.02$.

The third TGDM takes the central surface output Φ_{cent} as its initialization. We again apply an additional barrier constraint as in the previous algorithm to make sure that the outer surface stays outside of the central one. This barrier constraint is imposed by preventing the evolving pial surface level set function Φ_{out} from getting smaller than the initialization, Φ_{cent}. CCMC is again used to define the explicit pial surface mesh from the final Φ_{out} after convergence.

5.2.10 Cortical thickness and curvature

After the three surfaces are obtained, we can compute several properties of the segmented brain cortex such as the thickness of the cortex volume, and the curvature profile of the cortical surfaces. Here, we adopt a simple thickness measure, similar to that in [34]. At each grid point between the inner and outer surface, the thickness is defined to be the sum of the distances from that point to the inner and the outer surface. Note that at such a grid point, the signed distance function of the inner surface is positive and that of the outer surface is negative. Hence, the thickness map T is computed by:

$$T(\mathbf{x}) = \Phi_{\text{in}}(\mathbf{x}) - \Phi_{\text{out}}(\mathbf{x}).$$

To display thickness on the computed central surface, we use linear interpolation of this thickness field to determine thickness values on each node of the central surface mesh. We note that in [34], the thickness was computed on the outer surface using the absolute value of $\Phi_{\text{in}}(\mathbf{x})$. We also note that the Euclidean distance used here and in [34] may not be the optimal way to define cortical thickness. We would like to refer the reader to [32] and [173] for an alternative cortical thickness definition.

The mean and Gaussian curvatures of the reconstructed surfaces can also be calculated easily from their level set functions [34, 55]. For example, the mean curvature k_M can be computed from Φ using

$$\kappa_M = \frac{1}{2} \nabla \cdot \left(\frac{\nabla \Phi}{\|\nabla \Phi\|} \right)$$

$$= \frac{\sum_{(q,r,s)\in C}((\Phi_{qq} + \Phi_{rr})\Phi_s^2 - 2\Phi_q\Phi_r\Phi_{qr})}{2(\Phi_x^2 + \Phi_y^2 + \Phi_z^2)^{3/2}},$$

where $C = \{(x,y,z), (y,x,z), (z,x,y)\}$, and Φ_q and Φ_{qr} etc denote the first and second order partial derivatives respectively of Φ with respect to the subscripts.

5.3 Results and Discussion

Given the skull-stripped MR brain image and the two landmark points, our entire method currently takes less than 25 minutes on a desktop computer with a Linux operating system (2.2 GHz, Intel Pentium4 processor) to reconstruct all the three cortical surfaces. FANTASM requires 4 minutes 30 seconds. AutoFill takes less than 1 minute. The topology correction typically takes less than 2 minutes and the anatomically consistent GM enhancement requires less than 2 minutes. The TGDM for the inner surface takes less than 1 minute due to the close initialization. The TGDM for the central surface takes about 10 minutes, 6 minutes of which are spent for the computation of the gradient vector flow (GVF) force. The TGDM for the outer surface takes less than 4 minutes. There is still some room for improvement. For example, a multigrid method to solve the GVF PDE, (5.4), could potentially cut down the computation time by 4–5 minutes. Given that most algorithms currently report many hours to obtain similar results, we believe that our algorithm represents an important development for brain image analysis. We have applied the method to over a hundred MR brain images obtained from the Baltimore Longitudinal Study on Aging (BLSA) [174]. In the following we illustrate the performance of the method by presenting some results from its application to some BLSA data.

5.3.1 Qualitative evaluation

Figs. 5.14(a)–(c) show the reconstructed GM/WM, central, and pial surfaces, respectively, from a BLSA data set. Fig. 5.15–Fig. 5.17 show the reconstructed surfaces overlaying various cross sections of the original MR data. In particular, Fig. 5.15 shows several coronal slices of one brain data set and Fig. 5.16 shows several axial

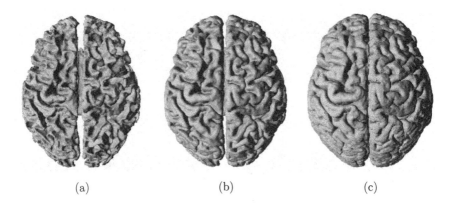

(a) (b) (c)

Figure 5.14: Top view of the reconstructed (a) GM/WM, (b) central, and (c) pial surfaces for one brain image.

slices of the same data set. Fig. 5.17 shows the coronal slices taken approximately at the anterior commissure (AC) of six different data sets, which correspond to the six subjects used in the landmark-error study described in the next subsection. From these figures, it can be seen that the estimated surfaces follow the folds of the cortex very well, including very narrow sulci. Subcortical structures are also being successfully separated from the brain cortex.

Although the cortical reconstruction results are accurate in general, some difficulties and inaccuracies still exist. For example, the cortical regions adjacent to the putamen structure are sometimes not segmented accurately due to the poor GM/WM contrast. As a result, the inner surface is often wrongly attached to the outer boundary of the putamen, as can be seen from Fig. 5.15(c) and Figs. 5.17(b) and 5.17(d) (as indicated by the arrows). This surface misplacement sometimes also happens near the posterior horns of the ventricle structure, as shown in Fig. 5.15(e) (as indicated by the arrow). Another weakness of the current method is that cortical structures around the brain stem area, e.g., the hippocampi structure, are not well preserved due to the AutoFill procedure. We are investigating further improvements in order to address these deficiencies.

We also ran a program to detect self-intersections on the final surface meshes,

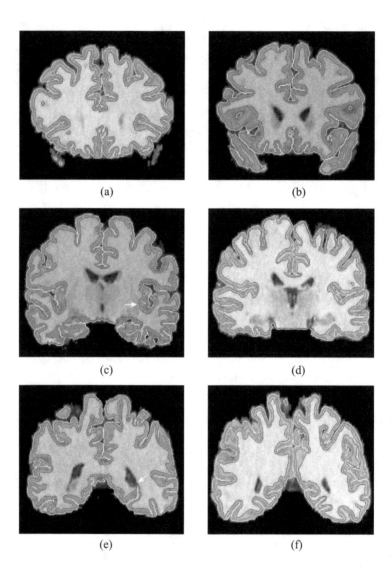

Figure 5.15: Coronal slices through an brain volume and the reconstructed surfaces (blue: inner; red: central; yellow: outer). (a)–(f): anterior to posterior.

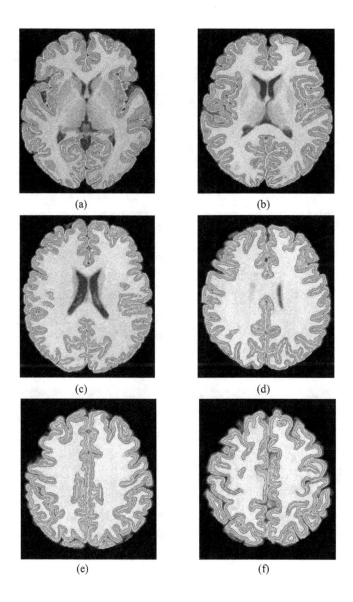

Figure 5.16: Axial slices through an brain volume and the reconstructed surfaces (blue: inner; red: central; yellow: outer). (a)–(f): bottom to top.

142

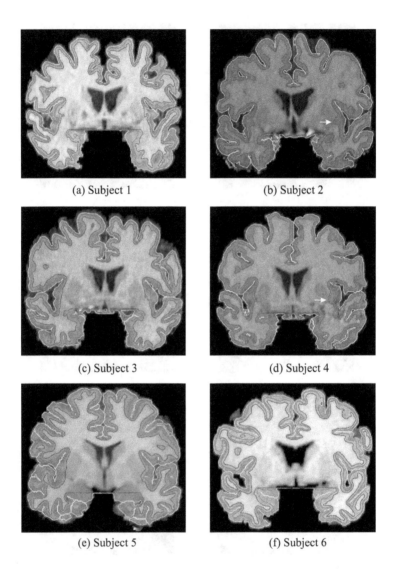

(a) Subject 1   (b) Subject 2

(c) Subject 3   (d) Subject 4

(e) Subject 5   (f) Subject 6

Figure 5.17: Coronal slices across the anterior-commissure of 6 brain volumes superimposed with the cross-sections of the corresponding reconstructed surfaces (blue: inner; red: central; yellow: outer).

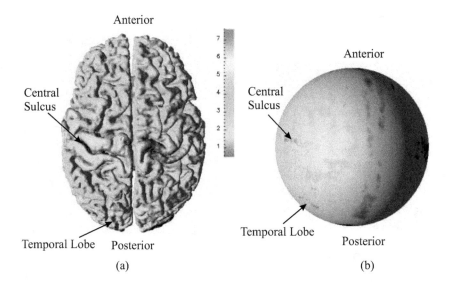

Figure 5.18: The thickness map shown on (a) the central surface and (b) the spherical map respectively.

and there are no self-intersections anywhere, as expected. In contrast, most cortical surface reconstructions obtained from parametric deformable models that do not explicitly prohibit them (cf. [36] and [35]) will have self-intersections. This is especially true for the pial surface, where many parts of the surface are essentially back-to-back in the tight sulci. The only other way to prevent (or reduce) self-intersections with parametric models is to increase the internal forces, which can have a very negative effect on the surface accuracy. Our method prevents self-intersections while simultaneously maintaining low internal forces to permit highly accurate (subvoxel) surface reconstructions.

Another important property of the method is that all the reconstructed cortical surfaces have the correct spherical topology, which were verified by checking the Euler number of the resulting surface meshes. With the guaranteed spherical topology, each surface is readily to be mapped to a sphere, which helps in visualizing geometrical or functional data on the cortex. We used the conformal mapping method described

144

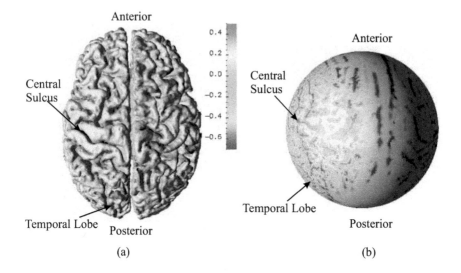

Anterior

Central
Sulcus

Temporal Lobe
Posterior

(a)

Anterior

Central
Sulcus

Temporal Lobe

Posterior

(b)

Figure 5.19: The curvature map shown on (a) the central surface and (b) the spherical map respectively.

in [29] to map the cortical surfaces to unit spheres. As the first example, Fig. 5.18 shows the cortical thickness map of one subject displayed both on the reconstructed central surface and on its spherical map. The thickness map is computed using the method described in Section 5.2.10. As we can see, the computed thickness mostly falls into the range of 1–5 mm, which agrees well with the literature [6–9]. Some abnormal values larger than 5 mm also exist, but they mainly occur around the brain stem area, where the cortical surfaces are not well defined. Another example is the mean-curvature map of the central surface as displayed in Fig. 5.19. As expected, the surface has large negative mean curvatures at the sulcal fundi and large positive curvature values at the gyral crowns. Thus, the mean curvature may be a useful feature for automatically tracing sulcal fundi on the reconstructed surface or parcellating the surface into sulcal and gyral regions [22, 175].

Table 5.1: Landmark errors on the central surfaces of 6 studies (in mm).

Landmark	\multicolumn{6}{c}{Subject}						Mean	Std
	1	2	3	4	5	6	Mean	Std
CS_1	1.14	2.20	1.00	0.13	0.09	0.67	0.87	0.78
CS_2	1.68	1.73	0.81	0.72	0.95	0.45	1.06	0.53
PCG_1	0.85	0.28	0.18	0.77	1.79	0.85	0.79	0.57
PCG_2	0.77	0.09	0.66	0.31	0.14	0.69	0.44	0.30
TLG_1	0.09	0.37	0.75	0.85	1.54	0.09	0.62	0.56
TLG_2	0.41	2.33	0.61	0.85	2.18	0.53	1.15	0.87
$CALC_1$	0.79	0.79	1.40	0.13	0.16	0.09	0.56	0.52
$CALC_2$	1.08	1.99	0.81	0.18	1.01	0.40	0.91	0.63
MFG_1	0.16	0.64	0.13	1.34	1.70	0.12	0.68	0.69
MFG_2	1.87	1.20	0.67	0.59	0.23	0.95	0.92	0.57
Mean	0.88	1.16	0.70	0.59	0.98	0.48	0.80	–
Std	0.59	0.84	0.37	0.40	0.79	0.31	–	–

5.3.2 Quantitative evaluation

To estimate the accuracy of the proposed method, we computed a set of landmark errors on six of the reconstructed central cortical surfaces, as shown in Table 5.1. The landmarks, ten on each brain, were manually picked on several major sulci and gyri (see [2]). As can be seen in the table, the errors are on the order of a voxel with a total average around 0.80 mm. For comparison purposes, we list in Table 5.2 the previously reported landmark error result [2], where the method used AFCM for segmentation, the median filtering for topology correction, a parametric deformable surface model, without using ACE. The new procedure exhibits both improved overall accuracy and substantially increased stability, as indicated by the lower standard deviation values. We believe that the improvement mainly comes from the better initialization made possible by the GTCA, and ACE. We note, however, that the landmarks were not designed specifically to test the robust of the algorithm with respect to the partial volume effect. More thorough validation of the cortical surface

146

Table 5.2: Landmark errors with the previous method [2] (in mm).

Landmark	Subject						Mean	Std
	1	2	3	4	5	6		
CS_1	1.21	2.40	1.48	0.22	0.63	0.47	1.10	0.80
CS_2	1.67	1.84	0.86	1.17	1.27	2.02	1.50	0.44
PCG_1	0.77	0.66	0.34	0.64	1.27	0.67	0.73	0.30
PCG_2	0.84	0.96	0.93	0.67	0.40	0.35	0.69	0.27
TLG_1	0.34	0.60	2.90	0.93	2.80	0.47	1.30	1.20
TLG_2	3.50	2.12	0.98	1.25	5.73	1.29	2.50	1.80
$CALC_1$	0.82	0.68	1.31	0.25	0.38	0.68	0.69	0.37
$CALC_2$	1.25	5.73	2.92	0.63	2.24	0.39	2.20	2.00
MFG_1	0.32	0.75	0.66	1.38	0.34	0.45	0.65	0.40
MFG_2	1.37	1.35	0.64	0.23	1.01	1.06	0.94	0.44
Mean	1.20	1.70	1.30	0.74	1.60	0.78	1.22	–
Std	0.91	1.60	0.91	0.43	1.70	0.53	–	–

reconstruction algorithm has been undertaken by other people in our research group, and the results will be reported elsewhere.

5.4 Summary

In this chapter, we have described a new approach for brain cortex segmentation that reconstructs all three key representative surfaces of the cortex. The method is computationally fast and robust, and produces surfaces that are geometrically accurate, have the correct topology, and do not self intersect or mutually intersect. The large automation and the full cortex characterization it provides makes it possible to conduct sophisticated neuroanatomical studies that involve large amount of imaging data.

Chapter 6

Moving Grid Geometric Deformable Models

Geometric deformable models are limited in accuracy and detail by the resolution of the computational grid used to solve the level set PDE. Thus, these methods may have difficulty in capturing the fine details that may be present in anatomical objects such as the tightly coupled pial surface of the cortex. Better accuracy and resolution generally requires the use of a finer computational grid, which typically causes an intolerable increase in required computation time and computer memory.

To address this issue, in this chapter we investigate the application of an adaptive grid technique within the framework of geometric deformable models (standard or topology-preserving). We show that the new *moving grid geometric deformable models* (MGGDMs) provide high accuracy while maintaining a low computational cost. We also show that the MGGDMs have the nice property of yielding a contour or surface with fewer nodes (vertices) than would be produced using a uniformly high-resolution grid. This contour or surface simplification property is highly desirable in practice because it facilitates post-processing computations. Although various surface simplification methods are available in the literature, they typically have problems in preserving the original surface topology and preventing the occurrence of surface self-intersections.

This chapter is organized as follows. We first introduce the resolution problem

148

in geometric deformable models, and motivate the need for the use of an adaptive grid (Section 6.1). We then summarize in Section 6.2 the principle of a particular adaptive grid method — specifically, the deformation moving grid method — and discuss its practical implementation. We also introduce a new grid nondegeneracy constraint to make sure that the computed grid map remains a one-to-one mapping and the grid does not have folding or overlapping. We describe the MGGDM method in Section 6.3, where the focus is placed on the design of grid adaptation criteria, and the design of suitable numerical methods to solve the transformed level set PDEs on the adaptive grid. Results are presented in Section 6.4 to demonstrate the benefit of using MGGDM. Finally, we summarize the chapter in Section 6.5.

6.1 Introduction

As introduced previously, geometric deformable models (GDMs) form a class of popular image segmentation tools that have been applied to a various of medical image segmentation problems. In the previous chapters, we developed a new geometric deformable model, TGDM, and successfully applied it to solve the cortical surface reconstruction problem. GDMs provide subpixel or subvoxel accuracy; but the level of accuracy is directly dependent on the size or resolution of the computational grid the model is implemented on. We call this the *resolution problem* of GDMs. The problem is common to all geometric deformable models and related to the implicit contour embedding scheme and its numerical implementation. The resolution problem is easy to understand: GDMs are governed by the solution of the level set PDE [cf. (2.10)], and the error in the numerical solution of the PDE depends on the resolution of the computational grid. In addition, as we mentioned in the introduction section of Chapter 4, the resolution of the computational grid also limits the level of details of the implicit contour that the model can reliably represent.

The problem is illustrated in Fig. 6.1. In Fig. 6.1(a), we show the ideal contour (green curves) overlaid on a computational grid. Unfortunately, the contour cannot be reliably represented at the given grid resolution level because different parts of the contour intersect with the same grid edge, as indicated by the two red arrows.

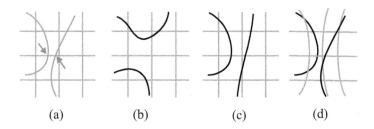

(a)   (b)   (c)   (d)

Figure 6.1: Resolution problem of level set methods. (a) Contours irrepresentable due to implicit embedding; (b) GDM changes topology; (c) TGDM keeps the contours separated by grid nodes; (d) An adaptive grid correctly resolves the desired contours.

With implicit contour embedding, the level set function will have the same sign at both ends of the edge, indicating that there are no contour intersections on the edge. Thus, if we apply a standard GDM to recover the truth contour, the result would most likely resemble Fig. 6.1(b), which has a totally different topology than that of the truth. The topology-preserving geometric deformable model (TGDM) introduced in Chapter 4 would shift one of the two curves in order to keep a grid point between them, as shown in Fig. 6.1(c). Although the topology is maintained, the accuracy is adversely affected.

One intuitive approach to overcome the resolution problem and improve the accuracy of GDMs is to use grid refinement. Uniform grid refinement typically leads to a large grid size and a low computational efficiency. Another class of approaches, called *adaptive grid techniques* [176], are known to be able to efficiently improve the numerical accuracy of solving partial differential equations while maintaining a relatively low computational cost. The approach that we investigate in this chapter falls into this category. As an intuitive illustration, Fig. 6.1(d) shows that a nonuniform adaptive grid with the same number of grid lines permits a faithful representation of the ideal contour.

Adaptive grid techniques are methods that locally refine or redistribute computational grid nodes according to a user-defined adaptivity criterion. Their importance and success have been amply demonstrated in the literature of numerical solutions for

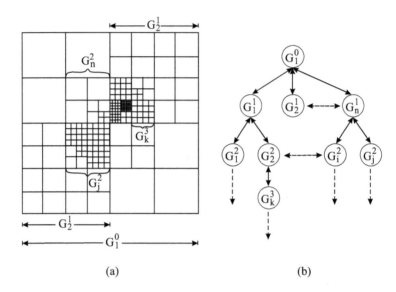

Figure 6.2: (a) Typical grid structure for local refinement methods, and (b) its tree representation.

PDEs [176]. However, the application of adaptive grid techniques within the GDM framework is still a new research area. Some additional research is necessary to study new requirements arising in GDMs and to design a fully consistent framework of adaptive grid GDMs, both standard and topology-preserving.

There are two competing adaptive grid techniques, the *local refinement method* and the *moving grid method*. In the local refinement method, additional grid nodes are inserted when and where they are needed, as illustrated in Fig. 6.2(a). This method requires a complicated hierarchical data structure to manage the many layers of grid nodes at different resolution levels [177], as illustrated in Fig. 6.2(b). The local refinement method has been used for quite some time in solving level set PDEs in computational physics [178, 179]; and a local refinement adaptive grid method has also been proposed for a special form of GDM [180]. The multiresolution approach in [45] where the grid is uniformly refined within the narrow band region, can also be viewed as a special case of the local refinement approach.

The second class of adaptive grid techniques is the *moving grid method*, which maintains a fixed uniform reference grid, but moves or reallocates the actual physical grid nodes according to an adaptivity requirement (cf. Fig. 6.3). The moving grid method has been applied previously in the computer vision literature for adaptive image reconstruction [181, 182]; however, it has been largely overlooked by the level set community, especially in the application to GDMs.

We found that local refinement methods are incompatible with the digital topology principles needed to implement the topology preservation constraint in TGDM. This is because the refined grid no longer has a uniform structure and the conventional digital topology principles no longer apply. In contrast, the uniform reference grid maintained by a moving grid method allows the same topology preserving principle to be applied as in the uniform grid case. In this work, we adopt a particular moving grid method, the *deformation moving grid method*, which was developed by Liao et al. over the past several years [183–186], and apply it to address the resolution problem of GDMs or TGDMs. The major reason for choosing this deformation moving grid method lies in the simplicity of its implementation, the ease of incorporating image information into the design of the adaptivity criterion, and its generality for arbitrary dimensions. The method is also one of few moving grid methods that theoretically guarantees no folding or overlapping in the final grid. (We note that grid folding can still happen in practice due to numerical errors; thus, in a later section, we introduce an additional nondegeneracy constraint to ensure the unfoldedness of the computational grid).

In the following presentation, we focus mainly on the 2D case for clarity and notation convenience. Additional comments will be added where necessary to help clarify the 3D implementation. Equations important for the 3D implementation are also provided in the appendices of this chapter.

6.2 Deformation Moving Grid Method

In this section, we first summarize the overall principle underlying the *deformation moving grid method* developed by Liao et al. over the last decade [183–186] and then present a recent variant proposed by Cao et al. [187]. Next, we describe its practical implementation including a spectral method that is used to solve the Poisson equations associated with this method. We believe that the spectral solver is simpler and more efficient than the numerical methods suggested in the original papers. We then introduce an unfoldedness criterion that guarantees the nonsingularity of the final grid map.

6.2.1 Basic principles

The description in this subsection mainly follows the presentation of the cited references [183–187], but is rewritten for clarity and consistency with later adaptation to the GDM framework.

Consider a general 2D time-dependent PDE

$$u_t = L(u_x, u_y, u_{xx}, u_{yy}, u_{xy}), \qquad (6.1)$$

which is defined on a rectangular physical domain $\Omega = [0,a] \times [0,b]$, where $L(\cdot)$ denotes a general function of the various spatial derivatives of the unknown function u. u_t, u_x, u_{xx}, etc. denote the partial derivatives of $u(x,y,t)$ with respect to the independent variable(s) indicated in the subscript(s); double subscripts denote second order partial derivatives. The level set PDE of GDMs (cf. (2.10)) can be written in the above form, with the u being replaced by the level set function Φ, and Ω being the domain of the image to be segmented.

Instead of uniformly refining the computational grid to improve the accuracy of solving (6.1), adaptive grid methods adaptively adjust the local grid structure in order to achieve the desired accuracy while maintaining a low computational cost. In partic-ular, the moving grid methods adaptively reallocate a fixed number of grid points on Ω to adjust the local grid resolution. Typically, the grid is locally condensed if $u(x,y,t)$ has rapid spatial variation, and the grid is coarsened if $u(x,y,t)$ changes smoothly. This grid reallocation is often described as a grid mapping $\mathbf{x} = \mathbf{x}(\boldsymbol{\xi}, t)$ from a certain reference domain Ω_r to the actual physical domain Ω as demonstrated in Fig. 6.3, where $\boldsymbol{\xi} = (\xi, \eta)$ $((\xi, \eta, \zeta)$ in 3D) denotes a point in Ω_r, and $\mathbf{x} = (x, y)$ $((x, y, z)$ in 3D)

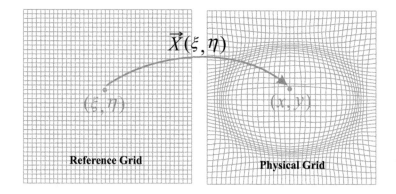

Figure 6.3: Adaptive grid generation with moving grid methods: the adaptive grid in the physical domain can be described as a mapping of the uniform reference grid.

is its image in the physical domain Ω. The reference domain Ω_r can be covered with a fixed uniform grid $\{ (\xi, \eta) \mid \xi = 0, \Delta\xi, \ldots, N_\xi \Delta\xi, \; \eta = 0, \Delta\eta, \ldots, N_\eta \Delta\eta \}$, where N_ξ and N_η denote the grid size, and $\Delta\xi$ and $\Delta\eta$ are the uniform grid spacing in the coordinate directions. The image of the reference grid under the mapping $\mathbf{x}(\boldsymbol{\xi}, t)$ then produces the adaptive physical grid. The time variable t simply indicates that the grid can be dynamically adapted to follow the evolution of the time-dependent PDE. Note that when Ω is a rectangular region as in our case, Ω_r is often identified with Ω or considered as a replica of Ω, and $\Delta\xi = a/N_\xi$ and $\Delta\eta = b/N_\eta$. A valid grid mapping $\mathbf{x}(\boldsymbol{\xi}, t)$ must be globally one-to-one so that grid tangling or overlapping does not exist.

Different moving grid methods differ in how to construct the grid mapping $\mathbf{x}(\boldsymbol{\xi}, t)$, and thus to control the adaptivity of the physical grid. The deformation moving grid method that we adopt here controls the grid adaptivity by specifying the Jacobian determinant $J(\mathbf{x})$ of the grid mapping:

$$J(\mathbf{x}) \triangleq \left| \frac{\partial \mathbf{x}}{\partial \boldsymbol{\xi}} \right| = 1/f(\mathbf{x}, t), \tag{6.2}$$

where $f(\mathbf{x}, t)$ is called the *monitor function*. Since the Jacobian determinant of the grid mapping is simply the ratio of the size of an area (volume in 3D) element in Ω

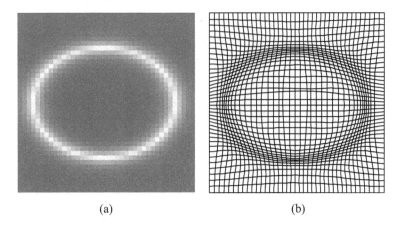

(a)   (b)

Figure 6.4: Example of a monitor function (a) and its corresponding adaptive grid (b).

and the size of its inverse image in Ω_r, (6.2) says that the size of a physical grid cell is inversely proportional to f. Therefore, the grid will be condensed in regions of high f values and coarsened where f is small, as illustrated in Fig. 6.4. In addition, by restricting $f(\mathbf{x}, t)$ to be positive and finite, $J(\mathbf{x})$ will be positive over Ω, and the grid is theoretically guaranteed not to fold onto itself. We note, however, that numerical errors in computing the grid mapping may easily ruin this property. It is therefore necessary to impose additional constraints during the numerical grid generation in order to prevent grid degeneracy; this will be discussed in detail in Section 6.2.3.

Because of (6.2), the grid adaptivity is fully determined by the choice of the monitor function. In the PDE literature, $f(\mathbf{x}, t)$ is typically chosen as a function of u and its derivatives. In a later section, we will discuss how to properly design the monitor function when applying the adaptive grid method to solve the level set PDEs in geometric deformable models.

Directly solving the grid mapping $\mathbf{x}(\boldsymbol{\xi}, t)$ from the Jacobian condition (6.2) is difficult and impractical because it leads to a highly nonlinear system of differential equations [188]. Instead, the deformation moving grid method considers the grid generation as a deformation process that is driven by a suitable deformation velocity field. The grid mapping $\mathbf{x}(\boldsymbol{\xi}, t)$ can then be computed by an integration of the velocity field, which we summarize here.

Let $\vec{v}(\mathbf{x}, t)$ denote the deformation velocity of the grid mapping, that is,

$$\vec{v}(\mathbf{x}, t) = \frac{D}{Dt}\mathbf{x}(\boldsymbol{\xi}, t),$$

where $\frac{D}{Dt}$ denotes the temporal derivative taken with the reference coordinates $\boldsymbol{\xi}$ being fixed, which corresponds to the so called *material derivative* in the literature of continuum mechanics [189]. A well-known identity in continuum mechanics gives the following relationship [189]:

$$\nabla \cdot \vec{v}(\mathbf{x}, t) = \frac{1}{J(\mathbf{x}, t)} \frac{DJ(\mathbf{x}, t)}{Dt}, \tag{6.3}$$

where $\nabla\cdot$ denotes the spatial divergence of the velocity field. This identity is called the *geometric conservation law* in Cao et al.'s paper [187]. Substituting (6.2) into (6.3) yields

$$\nabla \cdot \vec{v}(\mathbf{x}, t) = -\frac{1}{f(\mathbf{x}, t)} \frac{Df(\mathbf{x}, t)}{Dt},$$

or

$$f(\mathbf{x}, t)\nabla \cdot \vec{v}(\mathbf{x}, t) = -\frac{\partial f(\mathbf{x}, t)}{\partial t} - \vec{v}(\mathbf{x}, t) \cdot \nabla f(\mathbf{x}, t),$$

and finally,

$$\nabla \cdot (f(\mathbf{x}, t)\vec{v}(\mathbf{x}, t)) + \frac{\partial f(\mathbf{x}, t)}{\partial t} = 0. \tag{6.4}$$

(6.4) gives a necessary and sufficient condition that the deformation velocity field $\vec{v}(\mathbf{x}, t)$ must satisfy in order that the grid mapping $\mathbf{x}(\boldsymbol{\xi}, t)$ satisfies the Jacobian condition of (6.2).

From the theory of vector calculus, we find that the divergence condition (6.4) does not uniquely specify the solution $\vec{v}(\mathbf{x}, t)$. To resolve this lack of uniqueness, Liao et al. [183–186] specified the following condition

$$f(\mathbf{x}, t)\vec{v}(\mathbf{x}, t) = \nabla P(\mathbf{x}, t), \tag{6.5}$$

where $P(\mathbf{x},t)$ is an arbitrary potential function. Using (6.5) in (6.4) then leads to a simple Poisson equation that the potential function $P(\mathbf{x},t)$ must satisfy:

$$\nabla^2 P(\mathbf{x},t) = -\frac{\partial f(\mathbf{x},t)}{\partial t}. \tag{6.6}$$

Liao et al. [183–186] made an error, however, stating that the resulting mesh velocity field found by solving (6.5) is irrotational, and thus prevents excessive skewness of the adaptive grid. Actually, for the velocity field to be irrotational, one has to choose

$$\vec{v}(\mathbf{x},t) = \nabla P(\mathbf{x},t), \tag{6.7}$$

which is the approach taken in Cao et al.'s work [187]. We use the same symbol P for the potential function in both methods, but we will keep it clear which method we refer to. With the choice of (6.7) instead of (6.5), the resulting equation for the potential function $P(\mathbf{x},t)$ becomes more complicated:

$$\nabla \cdot (f(\mathbf{x},t)P(\mathbf{x},t)) = -\frac{\partial f(\mathbf{x},t)}{\partial t}. \tag{6.8}$$

This is still a Poisson equation, but one with spatially varying coefficients.

The above two Poisson equations [(6.6) and (6.8)] are solved under the Neumann boundary condition

$$\nabla P(\mathbf{x},t) \cdot \vec{N}(\mathbf{x}) = 0, \text{ for } x \in \partial\Omega,$$

where $\vec{N}$ denotes the normal vector at the boundary of the computational domain Ω. This condition makes sure that the computed grid mapping $\mathbf{x}(\boldsymbol{\xi},t)$ always maps the boundary of Ω_r to the boundary of Ω (since initially $\mathbf{x}(\boldsymbol{\xi},0)$ is the identity map), thus ensures that the physical grid covers the whole domain of Ω.

Given the monitor function $f(\mathbf{x},t)$ and following the above deformation strategy, the grid map $\mathbf{x}(\boldsymbol{\xi},t)$ can be computed in two steps. First the Poisson equation [(6.6) or (6.8)] must be solved and the deformation velocity $\vec{v}(\mathbf{x},t)$ computed. Then the grid map $\mathbf{x}(\boldsymbol{\xi},t)$ must be computed using a temporal integration of the velocity profile. We now discuss the numerical methods required for implementing each of the three steps.

6.2.2 Grid generation using the deformation moving grid method

We first assume that the grid map has been computed at time t_{k-1}, and we are to find the mapping at time t_k. t_{k-1} and t_k can be two consecutive time steps in discretizing (6.1), or can be just two dummy time instants when new adaptive grids are generated. The latter is the case we usually encounter when applying this method to the GDM framework. The monitor function $f(\mathbf{x}, t)$ is also assumed to be known at the two time instants t_{k-1} and t_k. Typically, at $k = 0$, the grid mapping $\mathbf{x}(\boldsymbol{\xi}, t_0)$ is assumed to be the identity map, i.e., $\mathbf{x}(\boldsymbol{\xi}, t_0) = \boldsymbol{\xi}$, and the monitor function is simply a constant function $f(\mathbf{x}, t_0) = 1$.

The deformation moving grid method finds the grid mapping at t_k by deforming the grid at t_{k-1}. This deformation process can be reparameterized independently of the original time-dependent PDE, especially when the grid generation is only performed sporadically, i.e., when t_{k-1} and t_k are two distant time steps in solving the original PDE. To emphasize this, we denote the reparameterization by another dummy variable τ, with $\tau \in (t_{k-1}, t_k]$. With this reparameterization, the monitor function also needs to be reparameterized between t_{k-1} and t_k. Linear interpolation is sufficient for this purpose, yielding

$$f(\mathbf{x}, \tau) = \frac{(\tau - t_{k-1})f(\mathbf{x}, t_k) + (t_k - \tau)f(\mathbf{x}, t_{k-1})}{t_k - t_{k-1}}, \text{ for } t_{k-1} < \tau \le t_k. \tag{6.9}$$

Using (6.9), the temporal derivative of the monitor function can be computed using

$$\frac{\partial f(\mathbf{x}, \tau)}{\partial \tau} = \frac{f(\mathbf{x}, t_k) - f(\mathbf{x}, t_{k-1})}{t_k - t_{k-1}}.$$

The grid mapping $\mathbf{x}(\boldsymbol{\xi}, t_k)$ at t_k is then computed in three major steps:

1. Solve for the scalar potential function $P(\mathbf{x}, \tau)$ for $\tau \in (t_{k-1}, t_k]$ from the Poisson equation:

$$\nabla^2 P(\mathbf{x}, \tau) = -\frac{f(\mathbf{x}, t_k) - f(\mathbf{x}, t_{k-1})}{t_k - t_{k-1}}, \tag{6.10}$$

   if using Liao et al.'s method or the equation

$$\nabla \cdot (f(\mathbf{x}, \tau)\nabla P(\mathbf{x}, \tau)) = -\frac{f(\mathbf{x}, t_k) - f(\mathbf{x}, t_{k-1})}{t_k - t_{k-1}}, \tag{6.11}$$

if using Cao et al.'s method. Both equations assume a Neumann boundary condition. Note that (6.10) is independent of τ, and needs only to be solved once for all τ. (6.11) needs to be solved repeatedly at different τ's due to the dependency of the coefficients $f(\mathbf{x}, \tau)$ on τ. Thus, as is discussed below, Cao et al.'s method is much slower than the original formulation by Liao et al.

2. Compute the deformation velocity $\vec{v}(\mathbf{x}, \tau)$ using

$$\vec{v}(\mathbf{x}, \tau) = \frac{\nabla P(\mathbf{x}, \tau)}{f(\mathbf{x}, \tau)}, \tag{6.12}$$

for Liao et al.'s method or

$$\vec{v}(\mathbf{x}, \tau) = \nabla P(\mathbf{x}, \tau), \tag{6.13}$$

for Cao et al.'s method.

3. Then, at each grid node indexed by the reference coordinates $\boldsymbol{\xi} = (\xi, \eta)$ $((\xi, \eta, \zeta)$ in 3D), solve the following ordinary differential equation (ODE) over τ by a proper numerical integration:

$$
\begin{aligned}
\frac{D}{D\tau}\mathbf{x}(\boldsymbol{\xi}, \tau) &= \vec{v}(\mathbf{x}(\boldsymbol{\xi}, \tau), \tau), \quad t_{k-1} < \tau \le t_k \\
\mathbf{x}(\boldsymbol{\xi}, \tau = t_{k-1}) &= \mathbf{x}_{t_{k-1}}(\boldsymbol{\xi}).
\end{aligned}
\tag{6.14}
$$

Implementation Considerations   There are several technical considerations in implementing the above algorithm that must be explained. First, in order for the Poisson equations to be solvable with the Neumann boundary condition, the integral of the source term in (6.10) or (6.11) must be zero (cf. [119]):

$$\int_{\Omega} \frac{f(\mathbf{x}, t_k) - f(\mathbf{x}, t_{k-1})}{t_k - t_{k-1}} d\mathbf{x} = 0, \text{ for all } k.$$

With the specification that $f(\mathbf{x}, t_0) = 1$, we must have

$$\int_{\Omega} [f(\mathbf{x}, t_k) - 1] d\mathbf{x} = 0, \text{ for all } k. \tag{6.15}$$

Therefore, any chosen monitor function must be normalized according to (6.15).

The second issue concerns the numerical solution of the Poisson equations [(6.10) and (6.11)]. The authors in [186] solve (6.10) using the successive over-relaxation (SOR) iterative method. The authors in [187] indicated that the SOR method can also be used to solve (6.11), but also proposed an alternative energy minimization formulation to directly compute the deformation velocity field $\vec{v}(\mathbf{x}, \tau)$, which is implemented using an FEM method. The authors acknowledged that the energy minimization with the FEM method is much more time consuming than solving the Poisson equation with the SOR method.

In our implementation, we propose to use spectral methods, which are known to be more efficient than the SOR method [190], to solve both types of Poisson equations. In particular, we apply the *discrete cosine transform* (DCT) method [190] to solve (6.10), which automatically takes into account of the Neumann boundary condition. Note that the DCT method requires discretizing (6.10) spatially on a rectilinear uniform computational grid. This grid can be chosen independently of the pre-specified reference grid. Usually, we use a grid two times as large in each dimension as the reference grid.

The equation (6.11) is much more difficult to solve, and we use an iterative spectral solver proposed very recently by Averbuch et al. [191]. This method iteratively solves a constant coefficient Poisson equation, with the final solution converging to that of the original equation. We apply the DCT solver at each iteration step. From our experience, this iterative spectral solver usually requires 6–8 iterations to converge in 2D, and around 15 iterations in 3D. In addition, since Cao et al.'s method requires solving (6.11) many times as τ changes, this method is in general much more computationally expensive and thus less practical than Liao et al.'s method, especially in the 3D case. But an advantage provided by Cao et al.'s method is that the adaptive grid it generates has much less skewness and the grid overlapping problem is less likely to happen. This tradeoff between grid quality and computation time is a dilemma in practice, and we are still looking for a better moving grid method, especially for 3D applications.

The third issue is related to the numerical integration of the grid equation, (6.14). Both explicit and implicit methods can be used to solve this ODE. For example, Liao et al. [186] suggested solving (6.14) using an implicit level set method. The advantage of using a level set method is not clear; besides, the implicit method produces the inverse mapping $\mathbf{x}^{-1}$, while the direct mapping $\mathbf{x}$ is needed for solving the original PDE. Thus, in our implementation, we apply the explicit Euler method to do the integration [190]. Note that to generate the adaptive computational grid, (6.14) need only be solved for a discrete set of $\boldsymbol{\xi}$'s, which correspond to the pre-specified uniform reference grid $\{\boldsymbol{\xi}_i = (\xi_i, \eta_i) \mid 1 \leq i \leq N_\xi N_\eta\}$, where $N_\xi N_\eta$ gives the reference grid size (again, we use the 2D case as an example).

To perform numerical integration of (6.14), τ also needs to be discretized in practice. We denote the discrete time steps by τ_j, where $\tau_j = j\Delta\tau$, $0 \leq j \leq N_\tau$, and $N_\tau = (t_k - t_{k-1})/\Delta\tau$. Then, the explicit temporal integration of (6.14) corresponds to updating the physical coordinates $\mathbf{x}(\boldsymbol{\xi}_i)$ for each grid node $\boldsymbol{\xi}_i$ by an increment equal to $\vec{v}(\mathbf{x}(\boldsymbol{\xi}_i, \tau_j), \tau_j)\Delta\tau$:

$$\mathbf{x}(\boldsymbol{\xi}_i, \tau_j) = \mathbf{x}(\boldsymbol{\xi}_i, \tau_{j-1}) + \vec{v}(\mathbf{x}(\boldsymbol{\xi}_i, \tau_{j-1}), \tau_{j-1})\Delta\tau, \quad 1 \leq i \leq N_\xi N_\eta, 1 \leq j \leq N_\tau. \quad (6.16)$$

The update is first performed for all grid nodes at fixed j, and then proceeds in time by replacing j with $j + 1$. In practice, we usually use $N_\tau = 10\text{--}20$ time steps to integrate (6.14). Note that the grid velocity is only available at uniformly sampled physical locations, which correspond to the uniform grid used by the spectral solver to solve the Poisson equations. Thus, interpolation is needed to get the velocity at the physical location $\mathbf{x}(\boldsymbol{\xi}_i, \tau_j)$ of each reference grid node $\boldsymbol{\xi}_i$ at a time instant τ_j. Linear interpolation is sufficient for this purpose.

6.2.3 Conditions for nondegenerate grids

Jacobian Positivity Condition and Its Discrete Analog. In order for the adaptive grid generated to be usable in solving the original time-dependent PDE, the grid must not be folded or have overlapping grid cells. This *nondegeneracy condition* requires that the grid mapping $\mathbf{x}(\boldsymbol{\xi}, t)$ (computed at any time t) be a global one-to-one map from the the reference domain Ω_r to the physical domain Ω. In the continuous formulation, a sufficient condition for the grid mapping to be one-to-one is that its

Jacobian determinant must be positive over the entire domain Ω_r. (Note that the Jacobian positivity only guarantees a local one-to-one mapping. A global one-to-one mapping is attained if both Ω_r and Ω are convex, and $\mathbf{x}(\boldsymbol{\xi}, t)$ maps the boundary of Ω_r to the boundary of Ω [192], which holds in our applications due to the image domain being always convex-shaped and the enforced Neumann boundary condition in the deformation moving grid method.)

In the cited references [183–186], the deformation grid method is claimed to guarantee the production of a valid grid mapping since it explicitly specifies the Jacobian determinants to be always positive. Unfortunately, in practice, numerical errors can easily ruin this property and cause grid folding or overlapping. In addition, in practice, the grid mapping is only computed at a discrete set of reference grid nodes, but not defined over the whole continuous domain. Thus, it is necessary to study the grid nondegeneracy condition in the discrete case, or in other words, to generalize the Jacobian positivity condition from the continuous case to the discrete one.

Such a generalization is presented in [193], where it is called the discrete analog of the Jacobian positivity condition. It is first assumed that a continuous grid mapping is obtained through a bilinear (trilinear in 3D) interpolation of its values given at the discrete set of grid nodes. This bilinear or trilinear interpolation assumption agrees with the usual practice of using finite difference operators to approximate the derivatives of the grid mapping. Under this assumption, the authors of [193] conclude that the grid mapping is guaranteed to be globally one-to-one if its discrete Jacobian determinants evaluated at each grid node are all positive.

To explain the condition more clearly, we consider first the 2D case and use Fig. 6.5 as an illustration. Consider the grid node with label $(1, 1)$ in the reference grid, located at the point O in the physical grid. By different combinations of forward and backward finite difference operators to approximate the derivatives of the grid mapping, at least four different Jacobian determinants can be computed at this grid node. For example, using the forward finite difference operator for both coordinate directions corresponds to evaluating the Jacobian determinant at O from the cell or quadrant $AODF$. The other three combinations give the Jacobian determinant computed from the other three cells (quadrants) that share O as a vertex. The discrete analog of the Jacobian

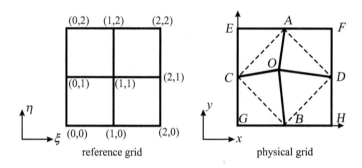

Figure 6.5: 2D reference and physical grid cells.

condition requires that all the four Jacobian determinants are positive. We note that the condition also ensures that the Jacobian determinant computed using the centered finite difference operator is positive, since it equals to an average of the previous four Jacobian determinants. Since the Jacobian determinants at O (e.g., the one computed from cell $AODF$) are simply the signed area of the triangles (e.g., triangle AOD) formed by O and two of its direct neighbors (4-neighbors), the discrete Jacobian condition actually enforces all the grid cells to remain convex, and thus grid folding or overlapping can never exist. Similarly, in the 3D case the discrete Jacobian condition requires all the Jacobian determinants evaluated at a grid node (eight if the node is not a boundary node) from each of the neighboring grid cells (octants) to be positive.

Enforcement of the Discrete Jacobian Positivity Condition within Deformation Moving Grid Method. Although the condition for a nondegenerate grid mapping is clear, it has not been discussed how to enforce this condition in a practical grid generation process such as the deformation moving grid method. We now present one approach.

The deformation moving grid method generates an adaptive physical grid by deforming an initially uniform grid. In the algorithm discussed in the previous section, each grid node is updated sequentially to a new physical location according to (6.16).

To satisfy the discrete Jacobian positivity condition and prevent the grid cells from folding, the movement of each grid node in the physical domain must be properly restricted. We now describe how to do this in both the 2D and 3D cases.

We first consider the 2D case. From Fig. 6.5, it is clear that moving grid node O can potentially change the Jacobian determinants evaluated both at its own location and at its four direct neighbors, A, B, C, and D. We first consider the Jacobian determinant at O computed from the cell $AODF$, whose value is simply the signed area of the triangle AOD. To avoid a sign change of the Jacobian determinant, O cannot move to the other side of the line AD. Given the deformation velocity $\vec{v}$ at O, denoted by $\vec{v}_O$, the time-of-flight, t_{AD}, for O to move across line AD can be simply computed using two inner products and a division, as follows

$$t_{AD} = \frac{\vec{N}_{AD} \cdot (\mathbf{x}_A - \mathbf{x}_O)}{\vec{N}_{AD} \cdot \vec{v}_O},$$

where $\vec{N}_{AD}$ denotes a vector normal to the line AD, which can be computed as

$$\vec{N}_{AD} = [y_D - y_A, -(x_D - x_A)]^T.$$

If $t_{AD} < 0$ then O does not cross line AD. If $t_{AD} > 0$ and $t_{AD} < \Delta\tau$ (the deformation step size), then the update by (6.16) will cause the Jacobian determinant at O to change sign. To prevent the sign change, we must restrict the movement of O by substituting $\Delta\tau$ in (6.16) with a value smaller than t_{AD}.

Similar analysis shows that O should not be allowed to cross the lines AC, BC, and BD either. That is, O must stay inside the convex hull formed by its 4-neighbors. We also need to consider the Jacobian determinants at the four 4-neighbors of O. Consider A, for example. The movement of O may cause the Jacobian determinant at A computed from either the quadrant $AECO$ or the quadrant $AODF$ to change sign. To prevent such sign changes, the movement of O must not cross the line AE or the line AF either.

The complete restriction on the movement of O is now clear: O cannot pass across the twelve lines, four from the convex hull $ACBD$ and eight from the grid edges formed by one 4-neighbor and one 8-neighbor, such as the lines AE, AF, CE,

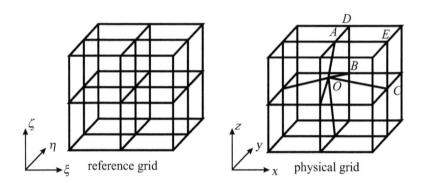

Figure 6.6: 3D reference and physical grid cells.

BH and etc. We modify the original deformation moving grid algorithm in the 2D case as follows: before updating the physical coordinates of a grid point O using (6.16), we first compute the twelve times-of-flight with respect to the twelve lines (the number of lines is reduced at a boundary node); we then take the minimum of all the non-negative time values and denote it by t_O. If t_O is bigger than $\Delta\tau$, then nothing need be changed. Otherwise, we substitute $\Delta\tau$ in (6.16) by $t_O - \epsilon$, where ϵ is a small positive number.

In the 3D case, the deformation of a grid node O must be restricted to avoid crossing thirty-two planes. Eight of the planes come from the convex hull formed by the 6-neighbors of O, for example, the plane passing through A, B, and C in Fig. 6.6. The remaining twenty-four planes are the planes passing through one 6-neighbor and two 18-neighbors, for example, the plane ADE. Again, given the deformation velocity $\vec{v}_O$ at the grid node, the time it takes for O to move across one such plane can be readily computed. Consider the plane ABC for example. We first compute a normal vector $\vec{N}_{ABC}$ of the plane as

$$\vec{N}_{ABC} = (\mathbf{x}_B - \mathbf{x}_A) \times (\mathbf{x}_C - \mathbf{x}_A).$$

The time, t_{ABC}, for O to move across the plane can then be computed as

$$t_{ABC} = \frac{\vec{N}_{ABC} \cdot (\mathbf{x}_A - \mathbf{x}_O)}{\vec{N}_{ABC} \cdot \vec{v}_O}.$$

In summary, to avoid grid folding in 3D, we compute the thirty-two times-of-flight, and take the minimum of all the non-negative values and denote it by t_O. The time-step size $\Delta\tau$ is then truncated to $t_O - \epsilon$ if initially $\Delta\tau \geq t_O$.

With the restriction on the grid node deformation, the generated physical grid is guaranteed to have no folding or cell overlapping. The bilinearly (trilinearly in 3D) interpolated continuous grid mapping $\mathbf{x}(\boldsymbol{\xi}, t)$ is thus guaranteed to be a homeomorphism from the reference domain to the physical domain, which then enables us to study the topology of the implicit contour(s) on the reference grid.

6.3 Moving Grid Geometric Deformable Model

In this section, we discuss the adaptation of the deformation moving grid method to the GDM framework. We focus on the design of the monitor function, and the development of new numerical schemes to compute the signed distance function and to solve the level set PDEs on an adaptive grid. We also discuss the design of a suitable isosurface algorithm when the adaptive grid method is applied. Our discussion generally applies to both the standard GDMs without the topology constraint and the topology-preserving ones. The differences in their implementation will be explicitly stated when necessary. We start with a discussion about the general framework of solving a time-dependent PDE with the moving grid technique. This helps explain the underlying principle and the special needs to successfully adapt the moving grid method to the GDM framework.

6.3.1 Solving time-dependent PDEs with the moving grid method

The original PDE, (6.1), is defined on the physical domain Ω. When a moving adaptive grid is used, the computational grid in the physical domain is no longer uniform. In order to simplify the numerical solution of the differential equation, the original equation must be first transformed to the reference domain Ω_r through the grid mapping; and then finite difference numerical methods can be applied to solve the transformed equation on the uniform reference grid.

We first consider the transformation of the spatial derivatives (we use the 2D case as an example, the corresponding equations for the 3D case are provided in Appendix 6.A). Let $U(\xi, \eta, t) = u(x(\xi, \eta, t), y(\xi, \eta, t), t)$. Applying the chain rule yields

$$
\begin{aligned}
U_\xi &= u_x x_\xi + u_y y_\xi \\
U_\eta &= u_x x_\eta + u_y y_\eta.
\end{aligned}
\tag{6.17}
$$

From (6.17), we can solve for u_x and u_y in terms of U_ξ and U_η as

$$
\begin{aligned}
u_x &= \frac{y_\eta}{J} U_\xi - \frac{y_\xi}{J} U_\eta \\
u_y &= -\frac{x_\eta}{J} U_\xi + \frac{x_\xi}{J} U_\eta,
\end{aligned}
\tag{6.18}
$$

where $J = x_\xi y_\eta - x_\eta y_\xi > 0$ is the Jacobian determinant of the grid mapping. Higher order derivatives such as u_{xx}, u_{yy}, and u_{xy} can be obtained similarly [176].

The time derivative must also be transformed, since u_t in (6.1) assumes that the physical coordinates (x, y) is fixed, not the reference grid (ξ, η). This transformation is found by applying the chain rule as follows

$$
\left(\frac{\partial U}{\partial t} \right)_{(\xi, \eta) \text{ fixed}} = \left(\frac{\partial u}{\partial t} \right)_{(x,y) \text{ fixed}} + \nabla u \cdot \mathbf{x}_t.
\tag{6.19}
$$

Substituting (6.19) into (6.1) yields

$$
U_t = L(u_x, u_y, u_{xx}, u_{yy}, u_{xy}) + \nabla u \cdot \mathbf{x}_t.
$$

We can then substitute all the partial derivatives with respect to the physical coordinates by partial derivatives with respect to the reference coordinates using relationships similar to (6.18), and arrive at a new PDE defined on the reference grid:

$$
U_t = \tilde{L}(U_\xi, U_\eta, U_{\xi\xi}, U_{\eta\eta}, U_{\xi\eta}) + \left(\frac{y_\eta x_t - x_\eta y_t}{J} U_\xi + \frac{x_\xi y_t - y_\xi x_t}{J} U_\eta \right).
\tag{6.20}
$$

This PDE can be solved using finite difference numerical schemes since the reference grid is a uniform rectilinear grid.

In the above derivations, the grid is assumed to deform continuously together with the temporal advancement of the time-dependent PDE. This pairwise solution is not necessary when solving the level set PDEs associated with GDMs, since it is unnecessary to get an accurate solution at every time step. This is one of the peculiarities we should take into consideration when applying the moving grid method. In particular, in our case grid adaptation need only be done sporadically. At times when the grid is held fixed, i.e., when $\mathbf{x}_t = 0$, the second term of the right-hand side of (6.19) and (6.20) disappears, and we need only solve

$$U_t = \tilde{L}(U_\xi, U_\eta, U_{\xi\xi}, U_{\eta\eta}, U_{\xi\eta}). \tag{6.21}$$

When grid adaptation is performed, we can assume that the physical evolution of the function $u(x, y, t)$ is stopped, i.e., $\tilde{L}(U_\xi, U_\eta, U_{\xi\xi}, U_{\eta\eta}, U_{\xi\eta}) = 0$, and only solve

$$U_t = \frac{y_\eta x_t - x_\eta y_t}{J} U_\xi + \frac{x_\xi y_t - y_\xi x_t}{J} U_\eta. \tag{6.22}$$

That is, we separate the temporal evolution of the original PDE from the sporadic grid adaptation.

To further illustrate this idea and for clarity, we change the time variable t in (6.22) to a dummy variable τ, which is consistent with the previous use of τ in describing the computation of the adaptive grid:

$$U_\tau = \frac{y_\eta x_\tau - x_\eta y_\tau}{J} U_\xi + \frac{x_\xi y_\tau - y_\xi x_\tau}{J} U_\eta. \tag{6.23}$$

(6.23) updates the physical function value associated with each reference grid node to reflect the change in the physical coordinates of the grid node. Another approach is to compute the functional value at the new grid locations using some interpolation procedure after the new grid is generated. By using (6.23) and solving it together with the grid generation equation, (6.14), we can avoid artifacts that might arise when applying a simple interpolation procedure. In addition, the topology-preserving constraint can be easily applied when solving (6.23) since it is in the form of a simple level set PDE, as will become clear below.

6.3.2   Moving grid GDM/TGDM algorithm

The level set PDE, (2.10), that is used in GDMs is a special case of the more general time-dependent PDE, (6.1). Therefore, the adaptive moving grid by deformation method can be directly applied. There are several facts that deserve special consideration, however. First, only the zero level set of the solution is of concern; therefore, the grid need only be refined near the zero level set and can be coarse otherwise. Correspondingly, the monitor function should resemble a delta function around the zero level set. Second, since only the final converged solution is of interest, it is not necessary to have an accurate solution for all time t. Thus, grid adaptation can be done sporadically, as mentioned in the previous subsection. Third, the level set function must be periodically reinitialized to be a signed distance function of its zero level set, as required in the traditional narrow band implementation of GDMs. The *fast marching method* (FMM) [55] usually used for this reinitialization, however, is no longer applicable in the adaptive grid case. In this subsection, we present the overall algorithm for the moving grid GDM/TGDM method. Then, in later subsections, we discuss how to accommodate the above considerations and address some other practical implementation issues. Again, we adopt the narrow band algorithm to implement the new adaptive grid GDMs, with or without the topology constraint.

In the following algorithm, we assume that the grid adaptation is performed each time the level set function is re-initialized as a signed distance function. For clarity, we present the algorithm in 2D, so that $\boldsymbol{\xi} = (\xi, \eta)$ denotes the fixed reference coordinates of a grid node and $\mathbf{x}(\boldsymbol{\xi}, t_k) = (x(\xi, \eta, t_k), y(\xi, \eta, t_k))$ denotes the actual physical coordinates of the grid node at the k-th adaptive grid. t_k is a pseudo time variable used to denote the time instant when the k-th adaptive grid is generated.

Algorithm 6.1 (Moving Grid Narrow Band Algorithm)

1. Set $k = 0$, $t_{k=0} = 0$, $f(\mathbf{x}, t_0) = 1$, and $\mathbf{x}(\xi, \eta, t_0) = (\xi, \eta)$ (the identity map). Initialize $\Phi(\xi, \eta, t_0)$ to be the signed distance function of the initial contour. Note that $\Phi(\xi, \eta, t_0)$ is the level set function evaluated at the physical location $(x(\xi, \eta, t_0), y(\xi, \eta, t_0))$.

2. If $k > 0$, re-initialize the level set function $\Phi(\xi, \eta, t_k)$ to be a signed distance function using the Fast Sweeping Method [194, 195] (see Section 6.3.4 for details).

3. Assume that the grid deformation is parameterized by τ, where $\tau \in (t_k, t_{k+1}]$.

   (a) Construct a new monitor function $f(\mathbf{x}, t_{k+1})$ from the signed distance function $\Phi(\xi, \eta, t_k)$ (see Section 6.3.3 for details).

   (b) Solve the moving grid Poisson equation, (6.10) if using Liao et al.'s method or (6.11) for Cao et al.'s method.

   (c) Compute the grid deformation velocity field $\vec{v}(\mathbf{x}, \tau)$ using (6.12) or (6.13), correspondingly.

   (d) Integrate the moving grid ODE, (6.14), for each grid node from $\tau = t_k$ until $\tau = t_{k+1}$ to get the new physical grid $\mathbf{x}(\xi, \eta, t_{k+1})$. The grid nondegeneracy condition proposed in Section 6.2.3 must be imposed here.

4. Advect the level set function to follow the grid motion. This is achieved by solving (6.23) with $U(\xi, \eta, \tau)$ replaced by $\Phi(\mathbf{x}(\xi, \eta, \tau), \tau)$ and using the initialization $\Phi(\xi, \eta, t_k)$, i.e., $\Phi(\mathbf{x}(\xi, \eta, t_k), t_k)$. The solution at $\tau = t_{k+1}$, $\Phi(\xi, \eta, t_{k+1})$, gives the level set equation sampled at the new physical grid $\mathbf{x}(\xi, \eta, t_{k+1})$. Note that (6.23) can be solved together with the integration of (6.14) in Step 3(d) to avoid the extra storage of the grid velocity (x_τ, y_τ).

5. Build the narrow band on the new grid $\mathbf{x}(\xi, \eta, t_{k+1})$ by finding all the reference grid nodes (ξ, η) such that $\Phi(\xi, \eta, t_{k+1})$ is within the narrow band range.

6. Transform (2.10) to the reference grid using the mapping $\mathbf{x}(\xi, \eta, t_{k+1})$. Advance the level set function $\Phi(\xi, \eta, t_{k+1})$ on the new grid $\mathbf{x}(\xi, \eta, t_{k+1})$ until reinitialization is required. If TGDM, the topology-preserving constraint is applied during every level set function update. Since (2.10) is first transformed to and then solved on the uniform reference grid (ξ, η), the simple point criterion check described in Chapter 4 for applying the topology constraint can be directly performed on the reference grid without any modification.

7. If the solution has not converged, set $k = k + 1$, and go to Step 2. Otherwise, stop.

6.3.3 Construction of the monitor function

We present two different schemes to define the monitor function for the moving grid GDMs. The first one makes the grid to follow the motion of the implicit contour, and the second one defines the monitor function directly based on the image to be segmented. The first scheme is more general and has been proposed in Liao et al.'s work [186]. When the second scheme is applicable, however, the adaptive grid need only be generated once beforehand, which drastically improves the efficiency of the overall moving grid GDM method. We assumed the first scheme when presenting the moving grid narrow band algorithm, Algorithm 6.1. The algorithm can be easily modified to accomodate the second scheme by performing the adaptive grid generation step only once at $k = 0$.

Monitor Function Design Based on the Level Set Function. As mentioned before, when solving the level set PDE, one only cares about the accuracy of the zero level set. Thus, a natural definition of the monitor function is [186],

$$f(\mathbf{x}) = \begin{cases} f_1 & \text{if } |\Phi(\mathbf{x})| \leq W; \\ f_2 & \text{if } |\Phi(\mathbf{x})| > W, \end{cases} \qquad (6.24)$$

where $f_1 > f_2$, $W > 0$ are user-defined constants that control the concentration of physical grid nodes around the zero level set. Since $\Phi(\mathbf{x})$ is the signed distance function of its zero level set, this monitor function creates fine grid cells around the zero level set and coarse cells otherwise. We note that $f(\mathbf{x})$ must be normalized according to (6.15).

This definition of the monitor function makes the grid nodes concentrate around the zero level set of the signed distance function. Since the zero level set keeps deforming, the grid has to be updated frequently to follow the evolution of the zero level set, as seen in Algorithm 6.1. Thus, this moving grid GDM scheme is far from efficient and has large redundancy, since in the application of deformable models one only cares about the accuracy of the final result, and all intermediate contours are rather useless.

Image-based Monitor Function Design. This second monitor function design provides a more efficient moving grid GDM algorithm. In image segmentation problems, GDMs are often designed to be attracted to salient image features such as locations of high image gradient. Thus, a proper computational grid should be condensed at desired image feature locations and coarsened otherwise. It may not be easy to come up with a construction that is suitable for all applications. However, for applications that rely on object boundary information, e.g., applications where the geodesic deformable model [46] is applicable, one can define the monitor function in a way similar to the definition of the metric term in the geodesic deformable model, for example,

$$f(\mathbf{x}) = 1 + \frac{|\nabla I_\sigma|^2}{K}, \tag{6.25}$$

where $|\nabla I_\sigma|$ is the gradient magnitude of the image (smoothed by a Gaussian filter with standard deviation σ), and K is a normalization factor. This monitor function provides fine grid cells at regions of high image intensity gradient, and coarse grids at homogeneous regions. The advantage of this monitor function design is that the adaptive grid is only generated once, significantly reducing the computation time of the method. Again, $f(\mathbf{x})$ must be normalized according to (6.15).

6.3.4 Distance transform on adaptive grids

Efficient computation of the signed distance function is an important part of GDM implementation. In a traditional uniform grid, the fast marching method (FMM) provides a very efficient approach to build the signed distance function from a given contour during both initialization and re-initialization steps. As introduced before, FMM is an $O(N \log N)$ algorithm which solves the following Eikonal Equation

$$\begin{aligned} |\nabla T(\mathbf{x})| &= 1 \text{ in } \Omega, \\ T &= 0 \text{ on } \Gamma, \end{aligned} \tag{6.26}$$

where Γ is the given contour.

When the moving grid is used, the above equation must be first transformed to the uniform reference grid so that finite difference numerical methods can be used.

172

By applying the transformation of (6.18), we get the transformed equation on the reference grid as (using the 2D case for illustration)

$$\frac{1}{J}\sqrt{g_{22}T_\xi^2 + g_{11}T_\eta^2 - 2g_{12}T_\xi T_\eta} = 1, \tag{6.27}$$

where $g_{11} = x_\xi^2 + y_\xi^2$, $g_{22} = x_\eta^2 + y_\eta^2$, $g_{12} = x_\xi x_\eta + y_\xi y_\eta$, and J is the Jacobian determinant as in (6.18). Unfortunately, (6.27) is no longer an Eikonal equation, and the FMM is no longer applicable.

Recently, there have been two methods proposed in the literature to solve the type of Hamilton-Jacobi equation appearing in (6.27): the *ordered-upwind method* by Sethian et al. [196] and the *fast sweeping method* by Tsai et al. [194, 195]. We chose to use the fast sweeping method to compute the signed distance function T in (6.27). Note that the fast sweeping method requires that the Hamiltonian is strictly convex, which in our case requires that $g_{11}, g_{22} > 0$ and $g_{11}g_{22} > g_{12}^2$. It can be proved that this condition is satisfied if and only if $J > 0$, which is guaranteed in our implementation of the deformation moving grid method.

The fast sweeping method uses an upwind and monotonic Godunov flux to approximate the Hamiltonian, and solves the equation by a Gauss-Seidel-type iterative algorithm with alternating sweeping directions. The computational complexity of the algorithm is $O(N)$, where N is the number of grid points at which the distance values are to be found. The details can be found in [194, 195].

6.3.5 Numerical schemes to solve the Level Set PDEs on adaptive grids

We now discuss the numerical schemes to approximate the transformed level set PDE on the reference grid. As in the case of a fixed uniform grid, different schemes are required to approximate the different types of force terms. Consider the general level set PDE of (2.10). The first term is the curvature force term. After transforming this term to the reference grid, we can approximate it using the centered finite difference scheme as in the traditional level set method, which involves the use of centered finite difference approximations to both the spatial derivatives of the level set function,

$\Phi_\xi, \Phi_\eta, \Phi_{\xi\xi}$, etc., and the derivatives of the grid mapping, x_ξ, x_η, y_ξ, and y_η.

The propagation force term $F_{\text{prop}}|\nabla\Phi|$ requires entropy-satisfying numerical schemes to avoid numerical instability such as oscillations. In a previous paper [67], we suggested the use of a *local Lax-Friedrichs* (LLF) scheme [197] to approximate $\nabla\Phi$ in this term. As known in the literature, the LLF scheme can be over-diffusive and often smoothes out fine details of the implicit contour. It is also tedious to generalize to the 3D case. We therefore designed an alternative method to approximate this propagation force term. The new scheme has been shown to work well through our experiments, but its convergence properties have not been rigorously analyzed. For clarity, we present the method in 2D here; the generalization to 3D is straightforward, and is presented in Appendix 6.B.

We note that on the reference grid, $|\nabla\Phi|$ has the following expression:

$$|\nabla\Phi| = \frac{1}{J}\sqrt{g_{22}\Phi_\xi^2 + g_{11}\Phi_\eta^2 - 2g_{12}\Phi_\xi\Phi_\eta}, \qquad (6.28)$$

where $g_{11}, g_{22}, g_{12}, g_{21}$, and J comes from the coordinate transformation, and are the same as in (6.27). We approximate the coordinate transformation terms by centered finite difference operators. To satisfy the entropy condition and ensure stability, the key is to choose suitable approximation to the partial derivatives of Φ with respect to the reference grid coordinates. We first denote the forward, backward, and centered difference operators in the two coordinate directions by $D^{+\xi}$ ($D^{+\eta}$), $D^{-\xi}$ ($D^{-\eta}$), and $D^{0\xi}$ ($D^{0\eta}$), respectively, and construct four upwind finite difference operators by taking into consideration the sign of F_{prop}, which is similar to what is proposed in the standard level set method [55]:

$$\begin{aligned}
D'^{+\xi}\Phi &= \text{sign}^+(F_{\text{prop}})(D^{+\xi}\Phi)^- - \text{sign}^-(F_{\text{prop}})(D^{+\xi}\Phi)^+, \\
D'^{-\xi}\Phi &= \text{sign}^+(F_{\text{prop}})(D^{+\xi}\Phi)^+ - \text{sign}^-(F_{\text{prop}})(D^{+\xi}\Phi)^-, \\
D'^{+\eta}\Phi &= \text{sign}^+(F_{\text{prop}})(D^{+\eta}\Phi)^- - \text{sign}^-(F_{\text{prop}})(D^{+\eta}\Phi)^+, \\
D'^{-\eta}\Phi &= \text{sign}^+(F_{\text{prop}})(D^{+\eta}\Phi)^+ - \text{sign}^-(F_{\text{prop}})(D^{+\eta}\Phi)^-,
\end{aligned} \qquad (6.29)$$

where $\text{sign}(\cdot)$ is 1 if the argument is positive and -1 otherwise, and $x^+ = \max(x, 0)$, $x^- = \min(x, 0)$.

Substituting Φ_ξ with either $D'^{+\xi}\Phi$ or $D'^{-\xi}\Phi$ and Φ_η with either $D'^{+\eta}\Phi$ or $D'^{-\eta}\Phi$ into (6.28) will give us four different evaluations of $|\nabla\Phi|$. We can also compute a fifth value of $|\nabla\Phi|$ by substituting into (6.28) Φ_ξ with $D^{0\xi}\Phi$ and Φ_η with $D^{0\eta}\Phi$. We finally take the maximum of all the five values as the value of $|\nabla\Phi|$ used in the computation of $F_{\text{prop}}|\nabla\Phi|$. This is the numerical scheme we currently applied to evaluate the propagation force term. In the 3D case, the computation of this force term involves the comparison of nine different evaluations of $|\nabla\Phi|$, as detailed in Appendix 6.B.

The next force term to approximate is the advection force term $\vec{F}_{\text{adv}} \cdot \nabla\Phi$. Since this force term is a linear term, a simple upwind approximation suffices. Again, consider the 2D case, and denote $\vec{F}_{\text{adv}} = (F_1, F_2)$. This term has the following form in the reference grid:

$$\vec{F}_{\text{adv}} \cdot \nabla\Phi = \frac{F_1 y_\eta - F_2 x_\eta}{J}\Phi_\xi + \frac{F_2 x_\xi - F_1 y_\xi}{J}\Phi_\eta.$$

Denote $a = (F_1 y_\eta - F_2 x_\eta)/J$ and $b = (F_2 x_\xi - F_1 y_\xi)/J$. The upwind approximation to this term can then be obtained as

$$\vec{F}_{\text{adv}} \cdot \nabla\Phi = a^- D^{-\xi}\Phi + a^+ D^{+\xi}\Phi + b^- D^{-\eta}\Phi + b^+ D^{+\eta}\Phi, \qquad (6.30)$$

where $a^+ = \max(a, 0)$, and $a^- = \min(a, 0)$ as in (6.29). We use the forward difference to compute the grid derivatives in a^+ and b^+, and the backward difference to compute a^- and b^-.

6.3.6   Advection of Φ during grid deformation

As discussed in Section 6.3.1 under (6.23), if we separate the grid deformation from advancing the level set equation, an extra interpolation is needed to update the level set function at each reference grid node to reflect the change in the physical coordinates. The interpolation can be replaced by an advection equation in the form of (6.23). The advantage is that we can apply the same upwind numerical scheme as above to get a more accurate solution than a simple interpolation scheme. Since (6.23) is just (2.10) with only the advection force term, the same topology preservation mechanism can also be applied to maintain the contour topology during this moving grid update.

Although the moving grid ODE, (6.14), is integrated over the whole reference grid, this advection equation need only be solved within a local region around the zero level set. The width of this local region should be larger than the expected largest grid displacement. We note that if this local update scheme is used, then another pass of the fast sweeping algorithm is required to get the signed distance values for each narrow band reference point.

6.3.7 Final contour extraction on an adaptive grid

The design of a proper isocontour or isosurface algorithm for the moving grid GDM is actually very easy. The uniform rectilinear reference grid allows the direct adoption of the connectivity consistent isocontour algorithm discussed in Chapter 3 to extract the final contour(s) from the level set function after convergence. The isocontour algorithm is performed on the reference grid, and is followed by an additional linear interpolation to find the physical coordinates of each contour node. Again, in the case of TGDM, since the topology constraint is enforced on the reference grid, the topology of the contour on the reference grid is guaranteed to be correct. In addition, since the grid mapping is guaranteed to be a homeomorphism, the physical contour is then homeomorphic to the reference-grid contour, and thus will also have the correct topology and have no self-intersections.

6.4 Results

In this section, we present several experiments to demonstrate the benefits of applying the moving grid method to GDMs. The results are mainly in 2D, but a preliminary result on 3D cortical surface reconstruction is also presented. The default implementation of the moving grid method follows Liao et al.'s approach because the grid generation is less time-consuming. It is explicitly stated when Cao et al.'s method is used instead.

6.4.1 2D experiments

Fig. 6.7(a) shows a phantom image comprising two circular cells. The initial contours for the deformable model are also shown as two dark curves. The image is of

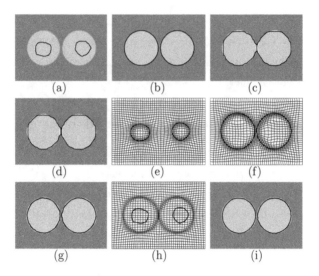

Figure 6.7: Segmentation of a phantom image. See text for details.

size 128×188. Using a computational grid of the same size, a TGDM with a signed pressure force and a curvature force produces the final boundary segmentation in Fig. 6.7(b). The topology constraint has no effect in this case since the two boundaries are well separated. The segmentation of Fig. 6.7(b) is used as the "ground truth" when comparing the results of later coarse grid segmentations.

We now choose a coarse computational grid of size 33×45 and apply both SGDM (i.e., GDM without the topology-preservation constraint) and TGDM with the same forces as before. The results of SGDM and TGDM segmentations are shown as dark curves in Fig. 6.7(c) and Fig. 6.7(d), respectively. The "ground truth" contours are also shown in the two figures as the white curves. Obviously, without the topology constraint, the two cells are wrongly merged. Both results have large errors as compared to the truth (the largest distance from the truth contour to either of the two coarse grid results is greater than 3 pixels). Figs. 6.7(e)–(g) illustrate the results when applying the moving adaptive grid. Figs. 6.7(e) and (f) show the deformed grid at an intermediate and the final stage together with its corresponding zero level set. The accuracy is improved, as shown in Fig. 6.7(g), where the final contours (dark curves) coincide well with the truth (white curves). The largest distance from the truth to the moving grid result is reduced to about 0.7 pixels. We note that the final contour in Fig. 6.7(g) comprises 146 vertices, which is comparable to the contours in Figs. 6.7(c) and 6.7(d), which have 130 and 136 vertices, respectively. In contrast, the "ground truth" contour in Fig. 6.7(b) has 542 vertices. In fact, the vertex reduction is roughly proportional to the reduction in grid lines in each direction. We note that if a local refinement adaptive grid or a multiresolution GDM implementation is used, the final contour will have similar size as the ground truth (if similar accuracy is maintained) since the effective computational grid in these methods are identical to a uniform grid as far as the deformable contour is concerned. Thus, in many applications, the moving grid GDM or TGDM implementation can have a strong advantage over the local grid refinement or multiresolution level set methods by yielding much smaller final contour size.

Fig. 6.7(h) shows the grid produced using the image derived monitor function [cf., (6.25)], which is created once before the contour evolution. Fig. 6.7(i) shows the final contours produced by this grid. The contours have only 142 vertices but are almost indistinguishable from the truth. The image derived grid adaptation requires solving the grid deformation equations only once, which improves the overall computational efficiency by another large factor.

In terms of computational speed, the time for generating the truth contour takes about 1.3s. SGDM or TGDM running on the uniform coarse grid takes about 0.2s. When the moving grid is applied, the computational time for each adaptive grid generation with Liao et al.'s method takes about 0.26s, which is almost equal to the time needed for the implicit contour propagation part (0.28s). Thus, the moving grid is more efficient if the grid generation only need be computed a very few number of times, as in the case of image-based grid generation. We also implemented Cao et al.'s method, which requires solving 10–20 varying-coefficient Poisson equations for generating one adaptive grid, and the solution of one varying-coefficient Poisson equation requires solving several constant-coefficients Poisson equations. It is typically more than 10 times slower than Liao et al.'s method in the 2D case and the final results

178

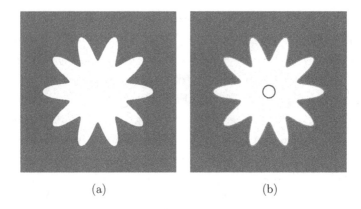

(a)   (b)

Figure 6.8: (a) A phantom image with a harmonic disk shaped object. (b) The initial
contour (blue curve) and the truth contour (red curve) overlaid on the original image.

are very similar. Thus, if Cao et al.'s method is used, the MGGDM can be much
slower than directly running GDM on the fine uniform grid. Thus, the method is
impractical unless a faster implementation can be found.

To get a more complete quantitative evaluation, we tested the algorithms using
a phantom image shown in Fig. 6.8. This image has a size of 512×512 pixels,
and consists of an object in the shape of a harmonic disk. We applied the geodesic
active contour model on several grids of different types and sizes, and compared the
accuracy and contour size of the final results, and also compared the computation
time. Topology-preservation is not an issue for this experiment, so we used SGDM.
To evaluate the accuracy of the results, we first ran SGDM with a uniform grid of
size 512×512 and took the resulting contour as the truth; this is shown as the red
curve in Fig 6.8(b). We then measured the errors of other results by computing the
distance from each vertices of the truth contour to the other contours. All the models
were initialized using a small circle inside the object, as shown as the blue curve in
Fig 6.8(b). When a moving grid GDM is applied, the adaptive grid was generated
only once using the monitor function definition of (6.25).

The results are summarized in Table 6.1, which is categorized into two groups,
uniform grid and adaptive grid. Rows 1–3 show the results of using uniform grids of

Table 6.1: Comparison of SGDM and MGGDM on grids of different type and size.

	Grid Size	Time (sec)	# Vertex	Maximum Error	Mean Error
Uniform Grid	256 × 256	5.88	1244	0.50	0.13
	128 × 128	2.35	624	1.71	0.33
	64 × 64	0.72	308	4.97	1.02
Adaptive Grid	256 × 256	14.8	1405	0.13	0.02
	128 × 128	5.22	812	0.42	0.05
	64 × 64	2.19	520	0.94	0.15

three different sizes. Rows 4–6 show the results when applying the moving adaptive grid method with different reference grid sizes. The grid sizes are shown in Column 2. Column 3 shows the total computation time, which includes the time for the grid generation when an adaptive grid is used. Column 4 shows the number of vertices in the final reconstructed contours. Columns 5 and 6 show the maximum error and the average error of each resulting curve as compared to the truth. The error is measured in the unit of the original image pixel size. As we can see, with the same grid type, a finer grid results in better accuracy, but also requires longer computation time. The more important comparison is across the two groups. For example, if we compare Row 6 with Row 2, we can see that the moving grid method allows the use of a much smaller grid size while achieving a much better accuracy in a comparable computation time. The resulting contour also has a smaller size when using the moving grid than using the uniform grid. If we use an even smaller grid as in Row 7 of the table, the moving grid GDM still achieves a comparable accuracy in average as the fine uniform grid. At the same time, the computation time is significantly reduced, and the final contour is further simplified.

In the last 2D experiment, we applied the moving grid GDMs to segment a real CT image of carpal bones. Fig. 6.9(a) shows the original image with the initial contours overlaid. The image is of size 151 × 220 pixels. We used a binary-flow GDM, which tries to separate the mean intensity of the region inside the evolving contour from

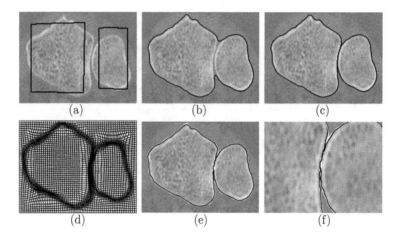

Figure 6.9: Segmentation of a carpal bone CT image. See text for details.

the mean of the outside. On a uniform grid of the same size as that of the image, SGDM produced the result in Fig. 6.9(b) and TGDM gave the result of Fig. 6.9(c). Due to the close adjacency of the two bones, SGDM created the wrong topology even at the finest grid. We then applied the moving grid TGDM with a reference grid of size 50×65. Fig. 6.9(d) shows the final physical grid together with the final contour segmentation. Fig. 6.9(e) displays this segmentation on the original image (dark curves), together with the "true" contours as in Fig. 6.9(c) (white curves). Fig. 6.9(f) is a magnified view at the gap between the two bone cells. Again, the two sets of contours are almost indistinguishable (the average distance is only 0.17 pixels in the unit of the original image), but the moving grid contours have only 290 vertices while the original grid contours have 838 vertices.

6.4.2 Moving grid TGDM for cortical surface reconstruction

The new moving grid geometric deformable model can potentially yield a better cortical surface reconstruction method, and make it feasible to process the super-high resolution brain images that have recently become possible. The research is still ongoing, and additional work is necessary to address the limitations of the current implementation, such as the long computation time. In the following, we present the result of a preliminary experiment, which applies the moving grid topology-preserving geometric deformable surface model to the cortical surface reconstruction problem and compares its performance against the uniform grid TGDM.

In this experiment, six brain images with manually picked central surface landmarks were used as the test data (cf. Section 5.3.2), but we upsampled the original images by a factor of two in each coordinate direction in order to simulate high-resolution brain images. Such an upsampling step is also desirable in practice in order to improve the accuracy of cortical segmentation. The original images all have a size of $256 \times 256 \times 198$, and after upsampling, the new images have size $512 \times 512 \times 396$. This large image size causes a huge increase in computation time and memory usage if the uniform grid TGDM implementation is used, as will be shown later. The resulting surface mesh also has a huge number of vertices, which can cause problem for post-processing steps, such as cortical unfolding or flattening, and surface-based data processing.

After upsampling, we apply the same cortical surface reconstruction procedure on the new images until the deformable surface reconstruction step. We then apply TGDM on three different computational grids to extract the central cortical surfaces. The first one uses a fine computational grid (the same size as the upsampled image). The second one uses a coarse computational grid of the original image size (a uniform grid of size $256 \times 256 \times 198$). The third one applies the moving grid TGDM method, where the reference grid is chosen to be the same as the coarse uniform grid (also with size $256 \times 256 \times 198$). The adaptive grid is computed only once before the surface deformation using Liao et al.'s deformation moving grid method, where the GM membership function is used as the monitor function so that the grid is condensed inside GM and coarsened otherwise. The image derived forces are computed initially on the fine uniform grid, and interpolated to the coarse uniform grid and the adaptive grid in the latter two TGDM implementations. After the central surfaces are reconstructed from all six studies using the three TGDM implementations, the landmark errors are then computed as a measurement of surface accuracy.

Fig. 6.10 first shows a visual comparison of the surface reconstruction results. It

182

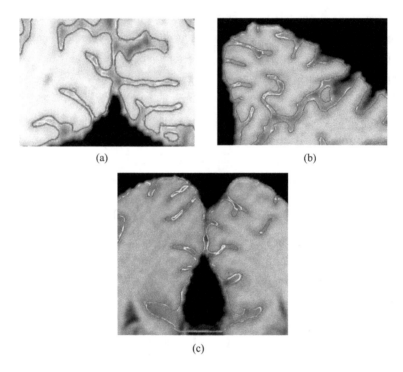

(a)   (b)

(c)

Figure 6.10: Magnified views of the central surface reconstruction results from three different TGDM implementations. Red: TGDM with fine uniform grid; yellow: TGDM with coarse uniform grid; blue: TGDM with adaptive grid.

Table 6.2: Performance comparison of TGDM with three different computational grids.

	Fine Uniform Grid	Coarse Uniform Grid	Moving Grid
Average Landmark Error	0.62 mm	0.94 mm	0.71 mm
Computation Time	45 minutes	4 minutes	28 minutes (10 for grid)
Memory Usage	1.2 GB	0.2 GB	0.5 GB
Mesh Size (vertices)	1,416,000	338,000	437,000

displays several magnified views of the reconstructed surfaces overlaid on 2D slices of the brain images, where the red, yellow, and blue curves correspond to the results from using the fine uniform grid, the coarse uniform grid, and the adaptive grid, respectively. As can be seen, the adaptive grid produces similar surface reconstruction results as the uniform fine grid, while the coarse grid surfaces differ quite significantly from the fine grid (and the adaptive grid) results and have obvious large errors within narrow sulcal regions.

Quantitative comparisons of using the three different grids are summarized in Table 6.2, which shows the overall average landmark error, the computation time, the memory usage, and the resulting surface mesh size (in average). The detailed landmark errors for each subject using the three computational grids are further plotted in Fig. 6.11. As we can see from Table 6.2 and Fig. 6.11, the fine uniform grid provides the best accuracy, that is, the smallest average landmark error. The computation time and memory usage is greatly increased, however. The resulting surface mesh is also huge, over four times the size of the coarse grid result. The coarse uniform grid gives the fastest computation and the smallest surface mesh, but the landmark error is much worse. The adaptive grid produces comparable landmark error as the fine uniform grid and the resulting surface mesh size is only slightly larger than that of the uniform coarse grid result. The computation time is yet unsatisfactory, however, and the time spent for the adaptive grid generation is already more than twice the total time required for uniform coarse grid TGDM. Thus, additional work is

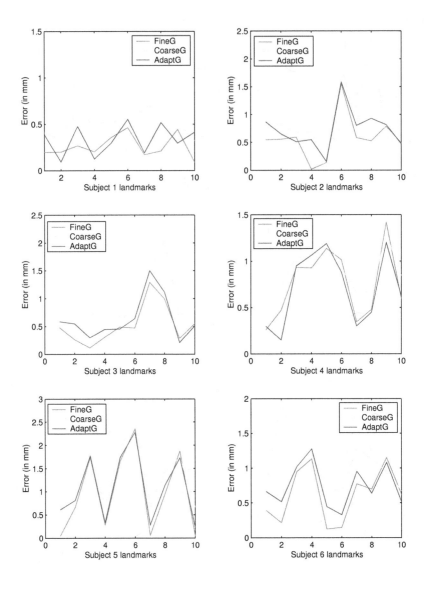

Figure 6.11: Landmark error comparison of central surface reconstructions using three different TGDM implementations. Red: TGDM on fine uniform grid; yellow: TGDM on coarse uniform grid; blue: TGDM on adaptive grid.

necessary to further optimize the moving grid TGDM implementation. In addition, we have observed that the deformation moving grid method has difficulty in producing a good adaptive grid to accommodate the complex shape of the brain cortex. The complex cortical geometry usually results in poor adaptive grid quality, including a large departure from orthogonality. Poor grid quality limits the accuracy of solving the level set PDE, a weakness that should be addressed in future work.

6.5 Summary

In this chapter, we adapted the deformation moving grid method to the framework of both standard and topology preserving geometric deformable models. We designed new numerical methods both for the implementation of the adaptive grid method and for solving level set PDEs on an adaptive grid. We also introduced a grid nondegeneracy constraint to make sure that the computed grid map has no folding or overlapping; and proposed an image based grid monitor function design, which further increases the efficiency of the overall method. As demonstrated by the experimental results, the grid adaptation increases the accuracy and efficiency of solving the level set PDEs associated with the geometric deformable models. Compared with the local refinement or multiresolution techniques, the moving grid method also provides an additional advantage of producing contours or surface meshes with fewer vertices, which can be a very significant advantage in 3D applications. Preliminary 3D experiments show that the new moving grid geometric deformable models can potentially help producing a better cortical surface reconstruction method. However, future research is necessary to fully evaluate the method and further improve its performance.

6.A   Transformation of Spatial Derivatives in 3D

Let $U(\xi, \eta, \zeta) = u(x(\xi, \eta, \zeta, t), y(\xi, \eta, \zeta, t), z(\xi, \eta, \zeta, t), t)$. Applying the chain rule yields

$$
\begin{aligned}
U_\xi &= u_x x_\xi + u_y y_\xi + u_z z_\xi \\
U_\eta &= u_x x_\eta + u_y y_\eta + u_z z_\eta \ , \\
U_\zeta &= u_x x_\zeta + u_y y_\zeta + u_z z_\zeta
\end{aligned}
\tag{6.31}
$$

which is the correspondence of (6.17) in the 3D case. From (6.31), we can solve for u_x, u_y, and u_z in terms of U_ξ, U_η, and U_ζ as

$$
\begin{aligned}
u_x &= \frac{1}{J}[(y_\eta z_\zeta - y_\zeta z_\eta)U_\xi + (y_\zeta z_\xi - y_\xi z_\zeta)U_\eta + (y_\xi z_\eta - y_\eta z_\xi)U_\zeta] \\
u_y &= \frac{1}{J}[(x_\zeta z_\eta - x_\eta z_\zeta)U_\xi + (x_\xi z_\zeta - x_\zeta z_\xi)U_\eta + (x_\eta z_\xi - x_\xi z_\eta)U_\zeta] \ , \\
u_z &= \frac{1}{J}[(x_\eta y_\zeta - x_\zeta y_\eta)U_\xi + (x_\zeta y_\xi - x_\xi y_\zeta)U_\eta + (x_\xi y_\eta - x_\eta y_\xi)U_\zeta]
\end{aligned}
\tag{6.32}
$$

where

$$
J = x_\zeta y_\xi z_\eta - x_\xi y_\zeta z_\eta - x_\zeta y_\eta z_\xi + x_\eta y_\zeta z_\xi + x_\xi y_\eta z_\zeta - x_\eta y_\xi z_\zeta
\tag{6.33}
$$

is the Jacobian determinant of the grid mapping $\mathbf{x}(\boldsymbol{\xi}, t) = (x(\xi, \eta, \zeta, t), y(\xi, \eta, \zeta, t), z(\xi, \eta, \zeta, t))$ in the 3D case.

In 3D, the advection equation, (6.23), is replaced by

$$
\begin{aligned}
U_\tau &= \nabla u \cdot \mathbf{x}_\tau \\
&= \frac{(y_\eta z_\zeta - y_\zeta z_\eta)x_\tau + (x_\zeta z_\eta - x_\eta z_\zeta)y_\tau + (x_\eta y_\zeta - x_\zeta y_\eta)z_\tau}{J} U_\xi \\
&\quad + \frac{(y_\zeta z_\xi - y_\xi z_\zeta)x_\tau + (x_\xi z_\zeta - x_\zeta z_\xi)y_\tau + (x_\zeta y_\xi - x_\xi y_\zeta)z_\tau}{J} U_\eta \ , \\
&\quad + \frac{(y_\xi z_\eta - y_\eta z_\xi)x_\tau + (x_\eta z_\xi - x_\xi z_\eta)y_\tau + (x_\xi y_\eta - x_\eta y_\xi)z_\tau}{J} U_\zeta
\end{aligned}
\tag{6.34}
$$

where the second equality is derived by applying (6.32) to the spatial derivatives of u in the term ∇u, and J is the same as in (6.33).

By applying the same transformation relationship to the Eikonal equation, (6.26), we get the transformed equation on the reference grid for the 3D case as

$$
\frac{F_{\text{prop}}}{J}\sqrt{g_{11}T_\xi^2 + g_{22}T_\eta^2 + g_{33}T_\zeta^2 - 2g_{12}T_\xi T_\eta - 2g_{13}T_\xi T_\zeta - 2g_{23}T_\eta T_\zeta} = 1,
\tag{6.35}
$$

where J is the same as in (6.33), and

$$
\begin{aligned}
g_{11} &= x_\zeta^2(y_\eta^2 + z_\eta^2) + (y_\zeta z_\eta - y_\eta z_\zeta)^2 - 2x_\eta x_\zeta(y_\eta y_\zeta + z_\eta z_\zeta) + x_\eta^2(y_\zeta^2 + z_\zeta^2), \\
g_{22} &= x_\zeta^2(y_\xi^2 + z_\xi^2) + (y_\zeta z_\xi - y_\xi z_\zeta)^2 - 2x_\xi x_\zeta(y_\xi y_\zeta + z_\xi z_\zeta) + x_\xi^2(y_\zeta^2 + z_\zeta^2), \\
g_{33} &= x_\xi^2(y_\eta^2 + z_\eta^2) + (y_\xi z_\eta - y_\eta z_\xi)^2 - 2x_\xi x_\eta(y_\xi y_\eta + z_\xi z_\eta) + x_\eta^2(y_\xi^2 + z_\xi^2), \\
g_{12} &= x_\zeta^2(y_\eta y_\xi + z_\eta z_\xi) + (y_\zeta z_\eta - y_\eta z_\zeta)(y_\zeta z_\xi - y_\xi z_\zeta) - x_\zeta[x_\xi(y_\eta y_\zeta + z_\eta z_\zeta) \\
&\quad + x_\eta(y_\xi y_\zeta + z_\xi z_\zeta)] + x_\xi x_\eta(y_\zeta^2 + z_\zeta^2), \\
g_{13} &= x_\eta^2(y_\xi y_\zeta + z_\xi z_\zeta) + (y_\xi y_\eta - y_\eta z_\xi)(y_\zeta z_\eta - y_\eta z_\zeta) - x_\eta[x_\zeta(y_\xi y_\eta + z_\xi z_\eta) \\
&\quad + x_\xi(y_\eta y_\zeta + z_\eta z_\zeta)] + x_\xi x_\zeta(y_\eta^2 + z_\eta^2), \\
g_{23} &= x_\xi^2(y_\eta y_\zeta + z_\eta z_\zeta) + (y_\xi z_\eta - y_\eta z_\xi)(y_\zeta z_\xi - y_\zeta z_\xi) - x_\xi[x_\zeta(y_\xi y_\eta + z_\xi z_\eta) \\
&\quad + x_\eta(y_\xi y_\zeta + z_\xi z_\zeta)] + x_\eta x_\zeta(y_\xi^2 + z_\xi^2).
\end{aligned}
\tag{6.36}
$$

Similar to the 2D case, (6.35) is a convex Hamilton-Jacobi equation if $J > 0$, and thus can be solved using a 3D version of the fast sweeping method [194, 195].

6.B Numerical Schemes to Solve Level Set PDEs on 3D Moving Grids

In this section, we present the numerical schemes to approximate the transformed level set PDE on the reference grid in the 3D case, which gives the 3D correspondence of the numerical schemes presented in Section 6.3.5. Same as in the 2D case, the curvature force term can be approximated using the standard centered finite difference scheme on the reference grid. Thus, in the following, we only discuss the numerical approximations to the propagation force term $F_{\text{prop}}|\nabla\Phi|$ and the advection force term $\vec{F}_{\text{adv}} \cdot \nabla\Phi$.

Propagation Force Term. Using the transformation relationship as given by (6.32), we obtain the following expression for the propagation force term on the reference grid:

$$
F_{\text{prop}}|\nabla\Phi| = \frac{F_{\text{prop}}}{J}\sqrt{g_{11}\Phi_\xi^2 + g_{22}\Phi_\eta^2 + g_{33}\Phi_\zeta^2 - 2g_{12}\Phi_\xi\Phi_\eta - 2g_{13}\Phi_\xi\Phi_\zeta - 2g_{23}\Phi_\eta\Phi_\zeta},
\tag{6.37}
$$

where J is the same as in (6.33), and g_{11}, g_{12}, and etc. are the same as in (6.36). We approximate the J and g's in this term by centered finite difference operators. To find the numerical approximation to the partial derivatives of Φ in (6.37), we first denote the forward, backward, and centered finite difference operators in the three coordinate directions by $D^{+\xi}$ ($D^{+\eta}$, $D^{+\zeta}$), $D^{-\xi}$ ($D^{-\eta}$, $D^{-\zeta}$), and $D^{0\xi}$ ($D^{0\eta}$, $D^{0\zeta}$), respectively, and then construct six upwind finite difference operators in analogy to (6.29):

$$
\begin{aligned}
D'^{+\xi}\Phi &= \operatorname{sign}^+(F_{\text{prop}})(D^{+\xi}\Phi)^- - \operatorname{sign}^-(F_{\text{prop}})(D^{+\xi}\Phi)^+, \\
D'^{-\xi}\Phi &= \operatorname{sign}^+(F_{\text{prop}})(D^{+\xi}\Phi)^+ - \operatorname{sign}^-(F_{\text{prop}})(D^{+\xi}\Phi)^-, \\
D'^{+\eta}\Phi &= \operatorname{sign}^+(F_{\text{prop}})(D^{+\eta}\Phi)^- - \operatorname{sign}^-(F_{\text{prop}})(D^{+\eta}\Phi)^+, \\
D'^{-\eta}\Phi &= \operatorname{sign}^+(F_{\text{prop}})(D^{+\eta}\Phi)^+ - \operatorname{sign}^-(F_{\text{prop}})(D^{+\eta}\Phi)^-, \\
D'^{+\zeta}\Phi &= \operatorname{sign}^+(F_{\text{prop}})(D^{+\zeta}\Phi)^- - \operatorname{sign}^-(F_{\text{prop}})(D^{+\zeta}\Phi)^+, \\
D'^{-\zeta}\Phi &= \operatorname{sign}^+(F_{\text{prop}})(D^{+\zeta}\Phi)^+ - \operatorname{sign}^-(F_{\text{prop}})(D^{+\zeta}\Phi)^-,
\end{aligned}
\tag{6.38}
$$

where $\operatorname{sign}(\cdot)$ is 1 if the argument is positive and -1 otherwise, and $x^+ = \max(x, 0)$, $x^- = \min(x, 0)$, the same as in (6.29).

Substituting Φ_ξ with either $D'^{+\xi}\Phi$ or $D'^{-\xi}\Phi$, Φ_η with either $D'^{+\eta}\Phi$ or $D'^{-\eta}\Phi$, and Φ_ζ with either $D'^{+\zeta}\Phi$ or $D'^{-\zeta}\Phi$, into (6.37) produces eight different evaluations of $F_{\text{prop}}|\nabla\Phi|$. We also compute a ninth value of $F_{\text{prop}}|\nabla\Phi|$ by substituting into (6.37) Φ_ξ with $D^{0\xi}\Phi$, Φ_η with $D^{0\eta}\Phi$, and Φ_ζ with $D^{0\zeta}\Phi$. We finally take the one value with the maximum magnitude as the final value of $F_{\text{prop}}|\nabla\Phi|$.

Advection Force Term. $\vec{F}_{\text{adv}}$ is a vector, and we denote it by $\vec{F}_{\text{adv}} = (F_1, F_2, F_3)$. After transforming the spatial derivatives of Φ to the reference grid, we get the following expression for the advection force term:

$$
\begin{aligned}
\vec{F}_{\text{adv}} \cdot \nabla\Phi &= \frac{(y_\eta z_\zeta - y_\zeta z_\eta)F_1 + (x_\zeta z_\eta - x_\eta z_\zeta)F_2 + (x_\eta y_\zeta - x_\zeta y_\eta)F_3}{J}\Phi_\xi \\
&+ \frac{(y_\zeta z_\xi - y_\xi z_\zeta)F_1 + (x_\xi z_\zeta - x_\zeta z_\xi)F_2 + (x_\zeta y_\xi - x_\xi y_\zeta)F_3}{J}\Phi_\eta , \\
&+ \frac{(y_\xi z_\eta - y_\eta z_\xi)F_1 + (x_\eta z_\xi - x_\xi z_\eta)F_2 + (x_\xi y_\eta - x_\eta y_\xi)F_3}{J}\Phi_\zeta
\end{aligned}
\tag{6.39}
$$

where J is the same as in (6.33). Denote

$$
\begin{aligned}
a &= \frac{(y_\eta z_\zeta - y_\zeta z_\eta)F_1 + (x_\zeta z_\eta - x_\eta z_\zeta)F_2 + (x_\eta y_\zeta - x_\zeta y_\eta)F_3}{J}, \\
b &= \frac{(y_\zeta z_\xi - y_\xi z_\zeta)F_1 + (x_\xi z_\zeta - x_\zeta z_\xi)F_2 + (x_\zeta y_\xi - x_\xi y_\zeta)F_3}{J}, \\
c &= \frac{(y_\xi z_\eta - y_\eta z_\xi)F_1 + (x_\eta z_\xi - x_\xi z_\eta)F_2 + (x_\xi y_\eta - x_\eta y_\xi)F_3}{J}.
\end{aligned}
\tag{6.40}
$$

The upwind approximation to the advection force term in 3D can be written as

$$
\begin{aligned}
\vec{F}_{\text{adv}} \cdot \nabla \Phi = \quad & a^- D^{-\xi}\Phi + a^+ D^{+\xi}\Phi + b^- D^{-\eta}\Phi + b^+ D^{+\eta}\Phi \\
& + c^- D^{-\zeta}\Phi + c^+ D^{+\zeta}\Phi
\end{aligned},
\tag{6.41}
$$

where $a^+ = \max(a,0)$, and $a^- = \min(a,0)$ as in (6.38), and similar for b^+, b^-, c^+, and c^-. We use the forward difference to compute the grid derivatives in a^+, b^+, and c^+, and the backward difference to compute a^-, b^-, and c^-.

We note that, in the 3D case, the advection equation, (6.34), is again in the form of a level set PDE with only the advection force term. Thus, an upwind numerical scheme similar to (6.41) can be used to approximate the right-hand side of (6.34).

191

Chapter 7

Conclusions and Future Work

This book concerned segmentation and boundary reconstruction in medical image processing. Several methods were developed to help produce accurate and anatomically consistent boundary localizations from medical images. Their merit has been demonstrated both by simulated experiments and by their successful application in an automatic, accurate, and anatomically consistent algorithm for cortical surface reconstruction from MR brain images. In this chapter, we summarize the main results of the book, and discuss potential directions for future research.

7.1 Multiscale, Graph-based Topology Correction Algorithm

In Chapter 3, we developed an automatic algorithm for removing topological defects both from binary volumes and from isosurfaces of general gray-scale or floating-point valued 3D images. The method, called GTCA, is useful both for the topology correction of an initial image segmentation or surface reconstruction with the wrong topology and for the generation of topologically correct initializations for topology-preserving deformable surface models. The formulation of GTCA uses techniques from digital topology, graph theory, isosurface generation, and mathematical morphology.

7.1.1   Main results

1. GTCA is intrinsically 3D and cuts (resp. fills) handles (resp. tunnels) naturally in arbitrary directions. It relies on rigorous digital topology principles, allows the use of any consistent pair of digital connectivity rules, and is guaranteed to find and remove all the handles (and tunnels).

2. GTCA removes handles locally, and does not make changes at regions with no handles. A foreground filter or background filter can be used alone to cut handles or fill tunnels exclusively, if desired.

3. GTCA can be applied to perform topology corrections on general isosurfaces computed from 3D gray-scale or floating-values images; the corrected isosurface exactly matches the original one except for necessary local topological corrections.

4. Experimental results show that GTCA can successfully correct the topology of WM segmentations with hundreds to thousands of handles, and the average number of voxels changed per handle is less than 3.5 in all the experiments.

5. Experimental results show that GTCA with an alternative B-F sequence produces the smallest volume change among all the tested sequences, and the average number of voxels changed per handle is less than 2.

6. Experimental results show that GTCA is a fast algorithm, and the topology correction typically takes less than 2 minutes on brain volumes of about $140 \times 200 \times 160$ voxels in size.

7.1.2   Future work

The current design criterion of GTCA aims solely to minimize the changes to the original volumes; the corrections GTCA makes may not necessarily follow anatomical boundaries as discussed in Chapter 3. It is conceivable that further improvements to the GTCA algorithm can be made by taking anatomical information into account.

For example, in the application to the cortical reconstruction problem, it would be desirable to incorporate either intensity information from the MR images or partial volume information from the fuzzy segmentation results into the algorithm. For such purposes, we might want to weight the voxels by a suitable function of the image intensity or the tissue membership function when performing the conditional topological expansion (CTE) and the cycle breaking. It may even be possible to develop a fully gray-scale topological correction scheme, rather than relying on a binary segmentation as in the current algorithm. More detailed anatomical information could also be applied, which may become available from higher-level image analysis steps such as a volumetric registration to a brain atlas. Such information would allow us to label sulci versus gyri, and even to label certain voxels as "anomalous" because they do not register well to labeled parts of the atlas. Such anomalous regions would then be made more susceptible to removal under topological correction.

In addition, there is an intriguing idea brought up in another independently developed topology correction algorithm [140], which suggests comparing the two potential corrections (cut or fill) for each handle and then making more intelligent choice than simply based on their size. This idea could be incorporated in the GTCA framework also in order to improve its performance. We can perform two topology corrections on a volume using either the foreground filter or the background filter exclusively, and then associate and compare the two corrections for each handle, and make the final choice based on the intensity information or other available anatomical knowledge.

Another direction of future research is to develop topology correction methods for other topological cases where the desired topology consists of one or more handles. For example, the human pelvis is an object that has two large handles. In these cases, we could apply GTCA with sequentially increasing scales until the genus of the corrected object matches the desired topology. This simple approach works if topological defects caused by image noise or other artifacts are known to have smaller scales than the "true" handles to be kept. It is in general a difficult problem, however, and may require the development of topology correction methods that can incorporate object shape information.

7.2 Topology-preserving Geometric Deformable Model

In Chapter 4, we proposed the incorporation of a topology constraint to the standard level set method, and derived the topology-preserving level set method (TLSM). The application of TLSM to the implementation of geometric deformable models led to the development of a new class of topology-preserving geometric deformable models (TGDM).

7.2.1 Main results

1. The implicit contour embedding scheme of traditional level set method was extended. It was demonstrated that the contour topology can be embedded in a binary fashion (digitally) while the continuous contour geometry can still be maintained.

2. Unlike traditional parametric deformable models, TGDM does not have the self-intersection problem and guarantees the valid manifold structure of the final contours (curves in 2D or surfaces in 3D).

3. Unlike traditional geometric deformable models, TGDM preserves the topology of the deforming contour(s), and guarantees the topological correctness of the final boundary segmentation results.

4. Theoretical analysis and experimental results show that TGDM shares similar convergence property as traditional deformable models, and is guaranteed to converge to a local constrained optimum.

5. Experimental results show that the proposed topology preservation scheme only incurs a small computational overhead, and the computational speed of TGDM is only 7% slower than that of SGDM.

7.2.2   Future work

Future work is required to address some remaining limitations of TGDM in order to further improve its performance. The first issue concerns the optimality of TGDM. As pointed out in Chapter 4, the outcome of TGDM can largely depend on its initialization due to the topology constraint. Although this problem is common to all existing deformable model methods and arises mainly because of the topology preservation requirement in medical image segmentation tasks, it is still desirable to find an approach that will achieve a (globally) optimal solution independent of the initialization. One approach, brought up in Chapter 4, would make use of a whole topology correction method as a projection operator to solve the constrained optimization problem of TGDM. Such a topology correction method, however, is not generally available for topological cases other than the spherical one.

The second issue is related to the first one, and lies in the fact that the current TGDM algorithm has little control over the final positions of the topological barriers produced that prevent topological changes from happening. Again, this is a problem also faced by the topology preserving parametric deformable models. To address this shortcoming, it may be necessary to design special forces that act only on the parts of the deforming contour that are declared as the topological barriers. Another worthwhile investigation is to explore the skeletal coupling idea of [1], in order to be able to predict the location where the topology barriers are going to form, and modify the original contour deformation scheme based on the prediction result.

The last overall concern about TGDM is related to the resolution problem brought up in Chapter 4, that is, TGDM cannot represent back-to-back curves or surfaces within one computational grid cell, as illustrated in Fig. 6.1. As a result, the topological barriers can only form around computational grid nodes. As discussed in Chapter 6, one possible approach to address this limitation is to make use of adaptive grid techniques; but a simpler approach that directly addresses this curve or surface representation problem may be desirable.

7.3 Brain Cortical Surfaces Reconstruction

In Chapter 5, we presented a systematic method for the reconstruction of three cortical surfaces from MR brain images. The method improves upon a previously developed method in our group [2] by incorporating the new topology correction algorithm and the new topology preserving geometric deformable model. Several new components were also designed to reduce the amount of manual interaction and to overcome the difficulty in reconstructing narrow sulcal folds. The new method is largely automatic, and provides a complete reconstruction of the brain cortex with high accuracy and topological correctness.

7.3.1 Main results

1. Experimental results show that the AutoFill method reliably separates most subcortical structures from the brain cortex. Only small parts of the putamen and the ventricle boundaries are occasionally attached to the inner cortical surface.

2. Experimental results show that the ACE method can successfully overcome the partial volume effect, and enables the central and the pial surfaces to accurately capture narrow sulcal folds.

3. Experimental results show that the proposed method can produce cortical surface reconstructions that are typically within 1 mm of the correct location throughout the cortex, and much more accurate than the previous approach [2] (0.80 mm versus 1.22 mm in average landmark error).

4. Experimental results show that the computed cortical thickness map mostly falls in the range of 1–5 mm, which is consistent with anatomical knowledge.

5. Experimental results show that the reconstructed cortical surfaces using the proposed method have no handles and no self-intersections.

7.3.2 Future work

Additional work is required to get a fully automatic cortical surface reconstruction procedure and further improve the accuracy and robustness of the overall method and its individual components. The current method requires manual intervention to help in removing non-brain tissues and picking two landmark points. Further investigation is necessary to eliminate such manual intervention by either developing new methods or incorporating some existing automatic methods proposed in the literature for specific purposes.

There is also room to further improve the accuracy and robustness of the current method. For example, the suggested improvements to the GTCA and the TGDM methods in the previous two sections can also help improve the performance of the overall cortical surface reconstruction procedure. The AutoFill method should be improved. The current algorithm is largely heuristic and over-simplified. A more elaborate algorithm should be designed to accurately delineate the boundaries of the ventricles and various subcortical structures. The accurate localization of these structures can further improve the accuracy of nearby cortical surfaces, and also provide useful information for various neuroscience studies.

Currently, only preliminary quantitative validations of the method have been performed. More comprehensive validation studies should be designed and conducted in order to fully evaluate the performance of the cortical surface reconstruction procedure and help optimize the various parameters for each individual component.

7.4 Moving Grid Geometric Deformable Model

In Chapter 6, we developed a class of moving grid geometric deformable models (MGGDMs) by incorporating a moving adaptive grid method into the framework of geometric deformable models, both traditional and the topology preserving ones. We studied in detail the deformation moving grid method, proposed new implementation schemes, and introduced a new nondegeneracy constraint to guarantee the correctness of the computed grid map. We also analyzed the special requirements for implement-

198

ing geometric deformable models on adaptive grids, proposed a new image based monitor function design, and suggested suitable numerical methods for computing signed distance functions and for solving general level set PDEs on adaptive grids.

7.4.1 Main results

1. A new nondegeneracy constraint was introduced to the original deformation moving grid method, which guarantees that the computed grid map is a one-to-one map and the adaptive grid has no folding or overlapping.

2. 2D experimental results show that the application of moving grid methods can efficiently improve the accuracy of geometric deformable models. It is shown that MGGDM on a coarse grid (128×128 in size) takes less time than SGDM on a fine grid (256×256 in size) (5.22s versus 5.88s), and gives an average segmentation error less than half of that of the SGDM method (0.05 pixels versus 0.13 pixels). With an even coarser computational grid (64×64 in size), MGGDM still produces comparable accuracy (average error = 0.15 pixels), but the computation time is largely reduced (2.19s versus 5.88s).

3. 2D experimental results show that MGGDM has the ability of achieving simultaneous contour simplification, and the reduction in the final contour size is approximately proportional to the reduction of the computational grid size in both dimensions.

4. 3D experimental results on six brain images show that MGGDM on a coarse grid produces comparable accuracy (landmark error = 0.71 mm on average) as SGDM on a fine computational grid (landmark error = 0.62 mm on average), but the memory usage is reduced by more than 50% (0.5 GB versus 1.2 GB) and the final surface mesh size is reduced by about 70% (437,000 vertices versus 1,416,000 vertices).

7.4.2 Future work

The computational speed is not yet satisfactory when applying the moving grid geometric deformable model in 3D. Both the adaptive grid generation procedure and the approach for solving level set PDEs on adaptive grids need to be further optimized. It would also help to investigate other choices of moving adaptive grid methods. As one disadvantage, the particular deformation moving grid method that we currently apply does not have direct control over the grid quality, such as grid orthogonality and smoothness. It is known that poor grid quality — for example, the departure from orthogonality or grid skewness — can limit the accuracy that can be gained when applying the moving grid method. Although the modification made by Cao et al. [187] partially overcomes the grid skewness problem, its implementation in 3D is extremely time-consuming. Such disadvantages should be addressed before the MGGDM method can be successfully applied to the cortical surface reconstruction or other 3D medical image segmentation tasks. Fortunately, the proposed MGGDM framework separates the adaptive grid generation step from the implementation of the model deformation, and should thus allow other alternative moving adaptive method to be easily incorporated.

7.5 Overall Perspective

The work presented in this book contributes to the field of image processing and medical image analysis through the development of new algorithms for performing boundary segmentation and surface reconstruction under topological and anatomical constraints. We hope that the research presented in this book may provide new insights in understanding the medical image segmentation problem and the challenges it poses, and help promote future development in the fields of image processing, signal processing, and medical imaging.

Bibliography

[1] T. B. Sebastian, H. Tek, S. W. Wolfe, J. J. Crisco, and B. B. Kimia, "Segmentation of carpal bones from 3D CT images using skeletally coupled deformable models," in *Proceedings of Medical Image Computing and Computer-Assisted Intervention (MICCAI)*. October 1998, pp. 1184–1194, Springer-Verlag.

[2] C. Xu, D. L. Pham, M. E. Rettmann, D. N. Yu, and J. L. Prince, "Reconstruction of the human cerebral cortex from magnetic resonance images," *IEEE Trans. Med. Imag.*, vol. 18, no. 6, pp. 467–480, 1999.

[3] Z. H. Cho, J. P. Jones, and M. Singh, *Foundations of Medical Imaging*, Wiley, New York, 1993.

[4] T. Kapur, W. E. L. Grimson, W. M. Wells III, and R. Kikinis, "Segmentation of brain tissue from magnetic resonance images," *Medical Image Analysis*, vol. 1, no. 2, pp. 109–127, 1996.

[5] D. G. Nishimura, *Principles of Magnetic Resonance Imaging*, Stanford University Press, Stanford University, 1996.

[6] C. von Economo, *The Cytoarchitectonics of the Human Cerebral Cortex*, Oxford Univ. Press, London, 1929.

[7] K. Zilles, *Cortex in the Human Nervous System*, Academic Press, San Diego, CA, 1990.

[8] L. D. Griffin, "The intrinsic geometry of the cerebral cortex," *Journal of Theoretical Biology*, vol. 166, no. 3, pp. 261–273, 1994.

[9] J. Beatty, *The Human Brain: Essentials of behavioral Neuroscience*, Sage Publications, Inc., California, 2001.

[10] A. M. Dale and M. I. Sereno, "Improved localization of cortical activity by combining EEG and MEG with MRI cortical surface reconstruction: A linear approach," *Journal of Cognitive Neuroscience*, vol. 5, no. 2, pp. 162–176, 1993.

[11] D. C. van Essen and H. A. Drury, "Structural and functional analyses of human cerebral cortex using a surface-based atlas," *Journal of Neuroscience*, vol. 17, no. 18, pp. 7079–7102, 1997.

[12] W. E. L. Grimson, G. Ettinger, T. Kapur, M. Leventon, W. Wells, and R. Kikinis, "Utilizing segmented MRI data in image-guided surgery," *Int. J. Patt. Recog. Artificial Intell.*, vol. 11, pp. 1367–1397, 1998.

[13] J.-F. Mangin, V. Frouin, I. Bloch, J. Regis, and J. Lopez-Krahe, "From 3D magnetic resonance images to structural representations of the cortex topography using topology preserving deformations," *Journal of Mathematical Imaging and Vision*, vol. 5, pp. 297–318, 1995.

[14] J. Talairach and P. Tournoux, *Co-planar Stereotaxic Atlas of the Human Brain*, Thieme Medical Publisher, Inc., Stuttgart, New York, 1988.

[15] H. A. Drury, D. C. Van Essen, C. H. Anderson, C. W. Lee, T. A. Coogan, and J. W. Lewis, "Computerized mapping of the cerebral cortex: A multiresolution flattening method and a surface-based coordinate system," *Journal of Cognitive Neuroscience*, vol. 8, no. 1, pp. 1–28, 1996.

[16] B. Fischl, M. I. Sereno, R. B. H. Tootell, and A. M. Dale, "High-resolution intersubject averaging and a coordinate system for the cortical surface," *Human Brain Mapping*, vol. 8, pp. 272–284, 1999.

[17] D. C. Van Essen, J. W. Lewis, H. A. Drury, N. Hadjikhani, R. B. H. Tootell, M. Bakircioglu, and M. I. Miller, "Mapping visual cortex in monkeys and humans using surface-based atlases," *Vision Research*, vol. 41, pp. 1359–1378, 2001.

[18] J. W. Phillips, R. M. Leahy, J. C. Mosher, and B. Timsari, "Imaging neural activity using MEG and EEG," *IEEE Engineering in Medicine and Biology*, vol. 16, pp. 34–42, 1997.

[19] D. L. Collins, G. Le Boualher, R. Benugopal, A. Caramanos, A. C. Evans, and C. Barillot, "Cortical constraints for non-linear cortical registration," in *Visualization in Biomedical Computing*, K. H. Hohne and R. Kikinis, Eds., Berlin, 1996, pp. 307–316, Springer.

[20] C. Davatzikos, "Spatial transformation and registration of brain images using elastically deformable models," *Comp. Vis. Image Understanding*, vol. 66, pp. 207–222, 1997.

[21] M. Vaillant and C. Davatzikos, "Hierarchical matching of cortical features for deformable brain image registration," in *Proceedings of the XVIth International Conference on Information Processing in Medical Imaging (IPMI'99)*, 1999, pp. 182–195.

[22] X. Tao, X. Han, M. E. Rettmann, J. L. Prince, and C. Davatzikos, "Statistical study on cortical sulci of human brains," in *Proceedings of the XVIIth International Conference on Information Processing in Medical Imaging (IPMI'01)*, M. F. Insana and R. M. Leahy, Eds. June 2001, LNCS 2082, pp. 475–487, Springer Verlag.

[23] P. Cachier, J. F. Mangin, X. Pennec, D. Rivière, D. Papadopoulos-Orfanos, J. Régis, and N. Ayache, "Multisubject non-rigid registration of brain MRI using intensity and geometric features," in *Proc. MICCAI 2001*, W. Niessen and M. Viergever, Eds., Berlin Heidelberg, 2001, LNCS 2208, pp. 734–742, Springer Verlag.

[24] P. Hellier and C. Barillot, "Cooperation between local and global approaches to register brain images," in *Proceedings of the XVIIth International Conference on Information Processing in Medical Imaging (IPMI'01)*, M. F. Insana and R. M. Leahy, Eds. 2001, LNCS 2082, pp. 315–328, Springer Verlag.

[25] G. J. Carman, H. A. Drury, and D. C. van Essen, "Computational methods for reconstructing and unfolding the cerebral cortex," *Cerebral Cortex*, vol. 5, pp. 506–517, 1995.

[26] B. Wandell, S. Engel, and H. Hel-Or, "Creating images of the flattened cortical sheet," *Investigative Ophthalmology and Visual Science*, vol. 36, pp. S612, 1996.

[27] S. Angenent, S. Haker, A. Tannenbaum, and R. Kikinis, "On the Laplace-Beltrami operator and brain surface flattening," *IEEE Trans. Med. Imag.*, vol. 18, pp. 700–711, 1999.

[28] B. Fischl, M. I. Sereno, and A. M. Dale, "Cortical surface-based analysis II: Inflation, flattening, and a surface-based coordinate system," *NeuroImage*, vol. 9, pp. 195–207, 1999.

[29] D. Tosun and J. L. Prince, "Hemispherical map for the human brain cortex," in *Proc. of SPIE Medical Imaging*, Feb 2001, vol. 4322, pp. 290–300.

[30] J. L. Tanabe, D. Amend, N. Schuff, V. DiSclafani, F. Ezekiel, D. Norman, G. Fein, and M. W. Weiner, "Tissue segmentation of the brain in Alzheimer disease," *Am. J. Neuroradiol.*, vol. 18, pp. 115–123, 1997.

[31] R. Kikinis, M. E. Shenton, G. Gerig, H. Hokama, J. Haimson, B. F. O'Donnell, C. G. Wible, R. W. McCarley, and F. A. Jolesz, "Temporal lobe sulco-gyral pattern anomalies in schizophrenia: An in vivo MR three-dimensional surface rendering study," *Neuro. Lett.*, vol. 182, pp. 7–12, 1994.

[32] S. E. Jones, B. R. Buchbinder, and I. Aharon, "Three-dimensional mapping of the cortical thickness using Laplace's equation," *Hum. Brain. Mapp.*, vol. 11, pp. 12–32, 2000.

[33] W. A. Edelstein, G. H. Glover, C. J. Hardy, and R. W. Redington, "The intrinsic signal-to-noise ratio in NMR imaging," *Magn. Reson. Med.*, vol. 3, pp. 604–618, 1986.

[34] X. Zeng, L. H. Staib, R. T. Schultz, and J. S. Duncan, "Segmentation and measurement of the cortex from 3d mr images using coupled surfaces propagation," *IEEE Trans. Med. Imag.*, vol. 18, pp. 100–111, 1999.

[35] D. MacDonald, N. Kabani, D. Avis, and A. C. Evans, "Automated 3-D extraction of inner and outer surfaces of cerebral cortex from MRI," *NeuroImage*, vol. 12, pp. 340–356, 2000.

[36] A. M. Dale, B. Fischl, and M. I. Sereno, "Cortical surface-based analysis I: Segmentation and surface reconstruction," *NeuroImage*, vol. 9, pp. 179–194, 1999.

[37] T. McInerney and D. Terzopoulos, "Deformable models in medical image analysis: A survey," *Medical Image Analysis*, vol. 1, no. 2, pp. 91–108, 1996.

[38] C. Xu, D. L. Pham, and J. L. Prince, "Medical image segmentation using deformable models," in *Handbook of Medical Imaging – Volume 2: Medical Image Processing and Analysis*, J. M. Fitzpatrick and M. Sonka, Eds., pp. 129–174. SPIE Press, May 2000.

[39] M. Kass, A. Witkin, and D. Terzopoulos, "Snakes: Active contour models," *Intl. J. Comp. Vision*, vol. 1, pp. 312–333, 1988.

[40] L. D. Cohen, "On active contour models and balloons," *CVGIP: Image Understanding*, vol. 53, pp. 211–218, 1991.

[41] T. F. Cootes, C. J. Taylor, D. H. Cooper, and J. Graham, "Active shape models – their training and application," *CVGIP: Image Understanding*, vol. 61, no. 1, pp. 38–59, 1995.

[42] C. Xu and J. L. Prince, "Snakes, shapes, and gradient vector flow," *IEEE Trans. Imag. Proc.*, vol. 7, no. 3, pp. 359–369, 1998.

[43] C. Chesnaud, P. Réfrégier, and V. Boulet, "Statistical region Snake-based segmentation adapted to different physical noise models," *IEEE Trans. Patt. Anal. Mach. Intel.*, vol. 21, pp. 1145–1157, 1999.

[44] V. Caselles, F. Catte, T. Coll, and F. Dibos, "A geometric model for active contours in image processing," *Numerische Mathematik*, vol. 66, pp. 1–31, 1993.

[45] R. Malladi, J. A. Sethian, and B. C. Vemuri, "Shape modeling with front propagation: A level set approach," *IEEE Trans. PAMI*, vol. 17, pp. 158–175, 1995.

[46] V. Caselles, R. Kimmel, and G. Sapiro, "Geodesic active contours," *International Journal of Computer Vision*, vol. 22, pp. 61–79, 1997.

[47] V. Caselles, R. Kimmel, G. Sapiro, and C. Sbert, "Minimal surfaces based object segmentation," *IEEE Trans. Patt. Anal. Mach. Intel.*, vol. 19, pp. 394–398, 1997.

[48] S. Kichenassamy, A. Kumar, P. Olver, A. Tannenbaum, and A. Yezzi, "Gradient flows and geometric active contours," in *Proc. ICCV'95*, Boston, USA, 1995, pp. 810–815.

[49] S. Kichenassamy, A. Kumar, P. Olver, A. Tannenbaum, and A. Yezzi, "Conformal curvature flows: From phase transitions to active vision," *Arch. Ration. Mech. Anal.*, vol. 134, pp. 275–301, 1996.

[50] A. Yezzi, S. Kichenassamy, P. Olver, and A. Tannenbaum, "A geometric snake models for segmentation of medical imagery," *IEEE Trans. Med. Imag.*, vol. 16, pp. 199–209, 1997.

[51] K. Siddiqi, Y. B. Lauziere, A. Tannenbaum, and S. W. Zucker, "Area and length minimizing flow for shape segmentation," *IEEE Trans. Image Proc.*, vol. 7, pp. 433–443, 1998.

[52] A. Yezzi, A. Tsai, and A. Willsky, "A statistical approach to snakes for bimodal and trimodal imagery," in *Proc. ICCV'99*, Corfu, Greece, 1999, pp. 898–903.

[53] N. Paragios and R. Deriche, "Geodesic active contours and level sets for the detection and tracking of moving objects," *IEEE Trans. Patt. Anal. Mach. Intel.*, vol. 22, no. 3, pp. 1–15, 2000.

[54] M. Leventon, E. Grimson, and O. Faugeras, "Statistical shape influence in geodesic active contours," in *Proc. IEEE Conf. CVPR'2000*, South Carolina, June 2000, pp. I:316–322.

[55] J. A. Sethian, *Level Set Methods and Fast Marching Methods*, Cambridge University Press, Cambridge, UK, 2nd edition, 1999.

[56] S. Osher and J. A. Sethian, "Fronts propagating with curvature-dependent speed: Algorithms based on Hamilton-Jacobi formulations," *J. Comput. Phys.*, vol. 79, pp. 12–49, 1988.

[57] T. McInerney and D. Terzopoulos, "Topologically adaptable snakes," in *Proc. ICCV'95*, 1995, pp. 840–845.

[58] H. Delingette and J. Montagnat, "New algorithms for controlling active contour shape and topology," in *European Conference on Computer Vision (ECCV'2000)*, Dublin, Ireland, 2000, pp. 381–395.

[59] X. Han, C. Xu, U. Braga-Neto, and J. L. Prince, "Graph-based topology correction for brain cortex segmentation," in *Proceedings of the XVIIth International Conference on Information Processing in Medical Imaging (IPMI'01)*, M. F. Insana and R. M. Leahy, Eds. June 2001, LNCS 2082, pp. 395–401, Springer Verlag.

[60] X. Han, C. Xu, U. Braga-Neto, and J. L. Prince, "Topology correction in brain cortex segmentation using a multiscale, graph-based algorithm," *IEEE Trans. Med. Imag.*, vol. 21, pp. 109–121, 2002.

[61] X. Han, C. Xu, and J. L. Prince, "A topology preserving deformable model using level set," in *Proc. of CVPR (CVPR'01)*, Hawaii, USA, December 2001, pp. II:765–770.

[62] X. Han, C. Xu, and J. L. Prince, "A topology preserving geometric deformable model and its application in brain cortical surface reconstruction," in *Geometric*

208

Level Set Methods in Imaging, Vision and Graphics, S. Osher and N. Paragios, Eds. Springer Verlag, New York, 2003.

[63] X. Han, C. Xu, and J. L. Prince, "A topology preserving level set method for geometric deformable models," *IEEE Trans. Patt. Anal. Machine Intell.*, vol. 25, pp. 755–768, 2003.

[64] X. Han, C. Xu, M. E. Rettmann, and J. L. Prince, "Automatic segmentation editing for cortical surface reconstruction," in *Proc. of SPIE Medical Imaging*, Feb 2001, vol. 4322, pp. 194–203.

[65] X. Han, C. Xu, D. Tosun, and J. L. Prince, "Cortical surface reconstruction using a topology preserving geometric deformable model," in *Proc. 5th IEEE Workshop on Mathematical Methods in Biomedical Image Analysis (MMBIA2001)*, Kauai, Hawaii, December 2001, pp. 213–220.

[66] X. Han, D. Pham, D. Tosun, M. Rettmann, C. Xu, and J. L. Prince, "CRUISE: Cortical reconstruction using implicit surface evolution," *NeuroImage*, vol. 23, pp. 997–1012, 2004.

[67] X. Han, C. Xu, and J. L. Prince, "A 2D moving grid geometric deformable model," in *Proc. of CVPR (CVPR'03)*, Madison, Wisconsin, June 2003, pp. I:153–160.

[68] J. C. Bezdek, L. O. Hall, and L. P. Clarke, "Review of MR image segmentation techniques using pattern recognition," *Medical Physics*, vol. 20, pp. 1033–1048, 1993.

[69] L. P. Clarke, R. P. Velthuzen, M. A. Camacho, V. Heine, L. O. Hall, R. W. Thatcher, and M. Silbiger, "MRI segmentation: Methods and applications," *Magnetic Resonance Imaging*, vol. 13, pp. 343–368, 1995.

[70] D. L. Pham, C. Xu, and J. L. Prince, "Current methods in medical image segmentation," *Annual Review of Biomedical Engineering*, vol. 2, pp. 315–337, 2000.

[71] A. F. Goldszal and D. L. Pham, "Volumetric segmentation of magnetic resonance images of the brain," in *Handbook of Medical Image Processing*, I. Bankman, Ed., pp. 185–194. Academic Press, San Diego, CA, 2000.

[72] C. K. Chow and T. Kaneko, "Automatic boundary detection of the left ventricle from cineangiograms," *Computers and Biomedical Research*, vol. 5, pp. 388–410, 1972.

[73] K. Wu, D. Gauthier, and M. D. Levine, "Live cell image segmentation," *IEEE Trans. Biomed. Eng.*, vol. 42, pp. 1–12, 1995.

[74] C. Lee, S. Hun, T. A. Ketter, and M. Unser, "Unsupervised connectivity-based thresholding segmentation of midsagittal brain MR images," *Computers in Biology and Medicine*, vol. 28, pp. 309–338, 1998.

[75] M. Sonka, V. Hlavac, and R. Boyle, *Image Processing, Analysis, and Machine Vision*, PWS Publishing, Pacific Grove, CA, 2nd edition, 1999.

[76] W. A. Barrett and B. S. Morse, "A relaxation algorithm for segmentation of the endocardinal surface from cine CT," in *IEEE Proc. Computers in Cardiology*, Jerusalem, Israel, 1989, pp. 95–98.

[77] P. M. J van der Zwet and J. H. C Reiber, "A new algorithm to detect irregular coronary boundaries: The gradient field transform," in *IEEE Proc. Computers in Cardiology*, Durham, NC, 1992, pp. 359–362.

[78] M. Sonka, M. D. Winniford, and S. M. Collins, "Robust simultaneous detection of coronary borders in complex images," *IEEE Trans. Med. Imag.*, vol. 14, pp. 151–161, 1995.

[79] I. N. Manousakas, P. E. Undrill, C. G. Cameron, and T. W. Redpath, "Split-and-merge segmentation of magnetic resonance medical images: Performance evaluation and extension to three dimensions," *Computers and Biomedical Research*, vol. 31, pp. 393–412, 1998.

[80] L. P. Clarke, R. P. Velthuizen, S. Phuphanich, and et al., "MRI: Stability of three supervised segmentation techniques," *Magnetic Resonance Imaging*, vol. 11, pp. 95–106, 1993.

[81] M. W. Vannier, C. M. Speidel, and D. L. Rickman, "Magnetic resonance imaging multispectral tissue classification," *News Physiol. Sci.*, vol. 3, pp. 148–154, 1988.

[82] M. X. H. Yan and J. S. Karp, "An adaptive Bayesian approach to three-dimensional MR brain segmentation," in *Information Processing in Medical Imaging*, Y. Bizais, C. Barillot, and R. D. Poala, Eds., Dodrecht, 1995, pp. 201–213.

[83] M. Kamber, R. Shinghal, D. L. Collins, G. S. Francis, and A. C. Evans, "Model-based 3-D segmentation of multiple sclerosis lesions in magnetic resonance brain images," *IEEE Trans. Med. Imag.*, vol. 14, pp. 442–453, 1995.

[84] W. E. Reddick, J. O. Glass, E. N. Cook, T. D. Elkin, and R. J. Deaton, "Automated segmentation and classification of multispectral magnetic resonance images of brain using artificial neural networks," *IEEE Trans. Med. Imag.*, vol. 16, pp. 911–918, 1997.

[85] G. Gerig, J. Martin, R. Kikinis, O. Kubler, M. Shenton, and F. A. Jolesz, "Unsupervised tissue type segmentation of 3D dual-echo mr head data," *Imag. Vis. Comput.*, vol. 10, pp. 349–360, 1992.

[86] M. E. Brandt, T. P. Bohan, I. A. Kramer, and J. M. Fletcher, "Estimation of CSF, white and gray matter volumes in hydrocephalic children using fuzzy clustering of MR images," *Comput. Med. Imaging Graph.*, vol. 18, pp. 25–34, 1994.

[87] Z. Liang, R. F. Jaszczak, and R. E. Coleman, "Parameter estimation of finite mixtures using the EM algorithm and information criteria with application to medical image processing," *IEEE Trans. Nuclear Sci.*, vol. 39, pp. 1126–1133, 1992.

[88] W. M. Wells, W. Grimson, R. Kikinis, and F. A. Jolesz, "Adaptive segmentation of MRI data," *IEEE Trans. Med. Imag.*, vol. 15, pp. 429–442, 1996.

[89] D. L. Pham and J. L. Prince, "An adaptive fuzzy c-means algorithm for images segmentation in the presence of intensity inhomogeneities," *Pattern Recognition Letters*, vol. 21, no. 1, pp. 57–68, 1999.

[90] D. L. Pham and J. L. Prince, "Adaptive fuzzy segmentation of magnetic resonance images," *IEEE Trans. Med. Imag.*, vol. 18, no. 9, pp. 737–752, September 1999.

[91] M. N. Ahmed, S. M. Yamany, N. Mohamed, A. A. Farag, and T. Moriarty, "A modified fuzzy c-means algorithm for bias field estimation and segmentation of MRI data," *IEEE Trans. Med. Imag.*, vol. 21, pp. 193–199, 2002.

[92] C. Baillard and C. Barillot, "Robust 3D segmentation of anatomical structures with level sets," in *Proc. MICCAI 2000*, S. L. Delp, A. M. DiGioia, and B. Jaramaz, Eds., Pittsburgh, USA, 2000, LNCS 1935, pp. 236–245, Springer.

[93] A. K. Jain, Y. Zhong, and S. Lakshmanan, "Object matching using deformable templates," *IEEE Trans. Patt. Anal. Machine Intell.*, vol. 18, pp. 267–278, 1996.

[94] A. K. Jain, Y. Zhong, and M. P. Dubuisson-Jolly, "Deformable template models: A review," *Signal Processing*, vol. 71, pp. 109–129, 1998.

[95] L. H. Staib and J. S. Duncan, "Boundary finding with parametrically deformable models," *IEEE Trans. Patt. Anal. Machine Intell.*, vol. 14, pp. 1061–1075, 1992.

[96] L. H. Staib and J. S. Duncan, "Model-based deformable surface finding for medical images," *IEEE Trans. Med. Imag.*, vol. 16, pp. 720–731, 1996.

[97] D. Terzopoulos and D. Metaxas, "Dynamic 3D models with local and global deformation: Deformable superquadrics," *IEEE Trans. Patt. Anal. Machine Intell.*, vol. 13, pp. 703–714, 1991.

[98] B. C. Vemuri, Y. Guo, C. M. Leonard, and S. H. Lai, "Fast numerical algorithms for fitting multiresolution hybrid shape models to brain MRI," *Med. Imag. Anal.*, vol. 14, pp. 637–645, 1997.

[99] M. Figueiredo, J. Leitao, and A. K. Jain, "Adaptive B-splines and boundary estimation," in *Proc. CVPR'97*, San Juan, PR, 1997, pp. 724–730.

[100] C. Nastar and N. Ayache, "Frequency-based nonrigid motion analysis: application to four dimensional medical images," *IEEE Trans. Patt. Anal. Machine Intell.*, vol. 18, pp. 1067–1079, 1996.

[101] U. Grenander, Y. Chow, and D. M. Keenan, *HANDS: A Pattern Theoretic Study of Biological Shapes*, Springer-Verlag, New York, 1991.

[102] M. I. Miller, G. E. Christensen, Y. Amit, and U. Grenander, "Mathematical textbook of deformable neuroanatomies," *Proc. Nat. Acad. Sci.*, vol. 90, no. 24, pp. 11944–11948, 1993.

[103] U. Grenander and M. I. Miller, "Computational anatomy: An emerging discipline," *Quart. Appl. Math.*, vol. LVI, pp. 617–694, 1998.

[104] P. M. Thompson and A. W. Toga, "A framework for computational anatomy," *Comput. Visual Sci.*, vol. 5, pp. 13–34, 2002.

[105] M. Mignotte, J. Meunier, and J.-C. Tardif, "Endocardial boundary estimation and tracking in echocardiographic images using deformable templates and markov random fields," *Patt. Anal. Appl.*, vol. 11, pp. 256–271, 2001.

[106] S. M. Pizer, D. S. Fritsch, P. Yushkevich, V. Johnson, and E. L. Chaney, "Segmentation, registration, and measurement of shape variation via image object shape," *IEEE Trans. Med. Imag.*, vol. 18, pp. 851–865, 1999.

[107] T. F. Cootes, A. Hill, C. J. Taylor, and J. Haslam, "Use of active shape models for locating structures in medical images," *Imag. Vis. Computing J.*, vol. 12, no. 6, pp. 355–366, 1994.

[108] G. Székely, A. Kelemen, C. Brechbühler, and G. Gerig, "Segmentation of 2-D and 3-D objects from MRI volume data using constrained elastic deformations of flexible fourier contour and surface models," *Med. Imag. Anal.*, vol. 1, pp. 19–34, 1996.

[109] N. Duta and M. Sonka, "Segmentation and interpretation of MR brain images: An improved active shape model," *IEEE Trans. Med. Imag.*, vol. 17, pp. 1049–1076, 1998.

[110] Y. Wang and L. H. Staib, "Boundary finding with prior shape and smoothness models," *IEEE Trans. Patt. Anal. Machine Intell.*, vol. 22, pp. 738–743, 2000.

[111] A. Hill, A. Brett, and C. Taylor, "Automatic landmark identification using a new method of non-rigid correspondence," in *Proc. XVth Intern. Conf. Info. Proces. Med. Imag. (IPMI'97)*, 1997, pp. 483–488.

[112] A. Hill, C. Taylor, and A. Brett, "A framework for automatic landmark identification using a new method of nonrigid correspondence," *IEEE Trans. Patt. Anal. Machine Intell.*, vol. 22, pp. 241–251, 2000.

[113] A. Frangi, D. Rueckert, J. Schnabel, and W. Niessen, "Automatic construction of multiple-object three-dimensional statistical shape models: Application to cardiac modeling," *IEEE Trans. Med. Imag.*, vol. 21, pp. 1151–1166, 2002.

[114] J. L. Lancaster, L. H. Rainey, J. L. Summerlin, and et al., "Automated labeling of the human brain: A preliminary report on the development and evaluation of a forward-transform method," *Human Brain Mapping*, vol. 5, pp. 238–242, 1997.

[115] G. E. Christensen, R. D. Rabbitt, and M. I. Miller, "3-D brain mapping using a deformable neuroanatomy," *Physics Med. Biol.*, vol. 39, pp. 609–618, 1994.

[116] S. Sandor and R. Leahy, "Surface-based labeling of cortical anatomy using a deformable atlas," *IEEE Trans. Med. Imag.*, vol. 16, pp. 41–54, 1997.

[117] T. McInerney and D. Terzopoulos, "Deformable models," in *Handbook of Medical Image Processing and Analysis*, I. Bankman, Ed., pp. 127–145. Academic Press, San Diego, CA, 2000.

[118] C. Xu, A. Yezzi, and J. L. Prince, "A summary of geometric level-set analogues for a general class of parametric active contour and surface models," in *Proc. of 1st IEEE Workshop on Variational and Level Set Methods in Computer Vision*, 2001, pp. 104–111.

[119] G. Strang, *Introduction to Applied Mathematics*, Wellesley Cambridge Press, 1986.

[120] J. A. Sethian, "A fast marching level set method for monotonically advancing fronts," *Proc. Nat. Acad. Sci.*, vol. 93, pp. 1591–1595, 1996.

[121] J. N. Tsitsiklis, "Efficient algorithm for globally optimal trajectories," *IEEE Trans. Automatic Control*, vol. 40, no. 9, pp. 1528–1538, 1995.

[122] H. Tek and B. B. Kimia, "Image segmentation by reaction-diffusion bubbles," in *Proc. Intl. Conf. Computer Vision*, Cambridge, MA, 1995, pp. 156–162.

[123] T. F. Chan and L. A. Vese, "Active contours without edges," *IEEE Trans. Image Proc.*, vol. 10, no. 2, pp. 266–277, 2001.

[124] D. Adalsteinsson and J. A. Sethian, "The fast construction of extension velocities in level set methods," *J. Comp. Phys.*, vol. 148, pp. 2–22, 1999.

[125] R. Goldenberg, R. Kimmel, E. Rivlin, and M. Rudzsky, "Fast geodesic active contours," *IEEE Trans. Image Proc.*, vol. 10, no. 10, pp. 1467–1475, 2001.

[126] J. Weickert, B. M. t. H. Romeny, and M. A. Viergever, "Efficient and reliable scheme for nonlinear diffusion filtering," *IEEE Trans. Image Proc.*, vol. 7, pp. 398–410, 1998.

[127] D. L. Chopp, "Computing minimal surfaces via level set curvature flow," *J. Comput. Phys.*, vol. 106, no. 1, pp. 77–91, 1993.

[128] D. Adalsteinsson and J. A. Sethian, "A fast level set method for propagating interfaces," *J. Comput. Phys.*, vol. 118, pp. 269–277, 1995.

[129] T. Y. Kong and A. Rosenfeld, "Digital topology: Introduction and survey," *CVGIP: Image Understanding*, vol. 48, pp. 357–393, 1989.

[130] A. Rosenfeld, "On connectivity properties of grayscale pictures," *Pattern Recog.*, vol. 16, pp. 47–50, 1983.

[131] G. Bertrand, "Simple points, topological numbers and geodesic neighborhoods in cubic grids," *Pattern Recognition Letters*, vol. 15, pp. 1003–1011, 1994.

[132] G. Bertrand, J. C. Everat, and M. Couprie, "Image segmentation through operators based on topology," *Journal of Electronic Imaging*, vol. 6, pp. 395–405, 1997.

[133] G. Malandain, G. Bertrand, and N. Ayache, "Topological segmentation of discrete surfaces," *Intl. J. Comp. Vision*, vol. 10, no. 2, pp. 183–197, 1993.

[134] L. Robert and G. Malandain, "Fast binary image processing using binary decision diagrams," *Comp. Vis. Image Understanding*, vol. 72, pp. 1–9, 1998.

[135] W. E. Lorensen and H. E. Cline, "Marching cubes: A high-resolution 3D surface construction algorithm," *ACM Computer Graphics*, vol. 21, no. 4, pp. 163–170, 1987.

[136] P. Ning and J. Bloomenthal, "An evaluation of implicit surface tilers," *IEEE Computer Graphics and Applications*, vol. 13, no. 6, pp. 33–41, 1993.

[137] B. K. Natarajan, "On generating topologically consistent isosurfaces from uniform samples," *Visual Computer*, vol. 11, no. 1, pp. 52–62, 1994.

[138] M. K. Agoston, *Algebraic Topology — A first course*, Marcel Dekker, Inc., New York, 1976.

[139] P. C. Teo, G. Sapiro, and B. A. Wandell, "Creating connected representations of cortical gray matter for functional MRI visualization," *IEEE Trans. Med. Imag.*, vol. 16, no. 6, pp. 852–863, 1997.

[140] N. Kriegeskorte and R. Goebel, "An efficient algorithm for topologically correct segmentation of the cortical sheet in anatomical MR volumes," *NeuroImage*, vol. 14, pp. 329–346, 2001.

[141] Z. Aktouf, G. Bertrand, and L. Perroton, "A 3D-hole closing algorithm," in *6th Int. Workshop on Discrete Geometry for Computer Imagery*, Lyon, France, 1996, pp. 36–47.

[142] F. Nooruddin and G. Rurk, "Simplification and repair of polygonal models using volumetric techniques," Technical Report 99-37, Georgia Inst. Tech., 1999.

[143] D. W. Shattuck and R. M. Leahy, "Topological refinement of volumetric data," in *Proc. of SPIE: Medical Imaging*, San Diego, USA, February 1999, vol. 3661, pp. 204–213.

[144] D. W. Shattuck and R. M. Leahy, "Topologically constrained cortical surfaces from MRI," in *Proc. of SPIE: Medical Imaging*, San Diego, USA, February 2000, vol. 3979, pp. 747–758.

[145] D. W. Shattuck and L. R. Leahy, "Graph based analysis and correction of cortical volume topology," *IEEE Trans. Med. Imag.*, vol. 20, pp. 1167–1177, 2001.

[146] Z. Aktouf, G. Bertrand, and L. Perroton, "A three dimensional hole closing algorithm," *Patt. Recog. Letter*, vol. 23, pp. 523–531, 2002.

[147] Z. Wood, H. Hoppe, M. Desbrun, and P. Schröder, "An out-of-core algorithm for isosurface topology simplification," *ACM Trans. Graphics*, vol. 23, pp. 190–208, 2004.

[148] B. Fischl, A. Liu, and A. M. Dale, "Automated manifold surgery: Constructing geometrically accurate and topologically correct models of the human cerebral cortex," *IEEE Trans. Med. Imag.*, vol. 20, no. 1, pp. 70–80, 2001.

[149] I. Guskov and Z. J. Wood, "Topological noise removal," in *Proceedings of Graphics Interface 2001*, 2001, pp. 19–26.

[150] G. Bertrand and G. Malandain, "A new characterization of three dimensional simple points," *Pattern Recognition Letters*, vol. 15, pp. 169–175, 1994.

[151] P. K. Saha and B. B. Chaudhuri, "Detection of 3D simple points for topology preserving transformations with application to thinning," *IEEE Trans. Patt. Anal. Mach. Intel.*, vol. 16, pp. 1028–1032, 1994.

[152] R. Sedgewick, *Algorithms in C*, Addison-Wesley, MA, 1990.

[153] G. P. McCormick, "Anti-zig-zagging by bending," *Management Science*, vol. 15, pp. 315–320, 1969.

[154] C. Pudney, "Distance-ordered homotopic thinning: A skeletonization algorithm for 3D digital images," *Computer Vision and Image Understanding*, vol. 72, no. 3, pp. 404–413, December 1998.

[155] H. K. Zhao, T. Chan, B. Merriman, and S. Osher, "A variational level set approach to multiphase motion," *J. Comput. Phys.*, vol. 127, pp. 179–195, 1996.

[156] L. C. Evans and R. F. Gariepy, *Measure Theory and Fine Properties of Functions*, CRC Press, Boca Raton, FL, 1992.

[157] M. S. Bazaraa and C. M. Shetty, *Nonlinear Programming: Theory and Algorithms*, John Wiley & Sons, New York, 1979.

[158] K. Siddiqi, A. Shokoufandeh, S. J.Dickinson, and S. Zucker, "Shock graphs and shape matching," *Int. J. Comput. Vision*, vol. 35, no. 1, pp. 13–32, 1999.

[159] K. Siddiqi, B. B. Kimia, A. R. Tannenbaum, and S. Zucker, "Shapes, shocks and wiggles," *Image Vis. Comput.*, vol. 17, pp. 365–373, 1999.

[160] J. Milnor, *Morse Theory*, vol. 51 of *Annals Math. Studies*, Princeton Univ. Press, New Jersey, 1963.

[161] B. T. Stander and J. C. Hart, "Guaranteeing the topology of an implicit surface polygonization for interactive modeling," in *Proc. SIGGRAPH'97*, 1997, pp. 279–286.

[162] D. W. Shattuck and R. M. Leahy, "BrainSuite: An automated cortical surface identification tool," *Med. Imag. Anal.*, vol. 6, pp. 129–142, 2002.

[163] C. Davatzikos and N. Bryan, "Using a deformable surface model to obtain a shape representation of the cortex," *IEEE Trans. Med. Imag.*, vol. 15, no. 6, pp. 785–795, 1996.

[164] M. Vaillant and C. Davatzikos, "Finding parametric representations of the cortical sulci using an active contour model," *Medical Image Analysis*, vol. 1, no. 4, pp. 295–315, 1997.

[165] M. Joshi, J. Cui, K. Doolittle, S. Joshi, D. Van Essen, L. Wang, and M. I. Miller, "Brain segmentation and the generation of cortical surfaces," *NeuroImage*, vol. 9, pp. 461–476, 1999.

[166] F. Kruggel and D. Y. von Cramon, "Measuring cortical thickness," in *Workshop on Mathematical Methods in Biomedical Image Analysis*, Los Alamitos, CA, 2000, pp. 154–161, IEEE Comp Soc.

[167] R. Goldenberg, R. Kimmel, E. Rivlin, and M. Rudzsky, "Cortex segmentation: A fast variational geometric approach," *IEEE Trans. Med. Imag.*, vol. 21, pp. 1544–1551, 2002.

[168] A. F. Goldszal, C. Davatzikos, D. L. Pham, M. X. H. Yan, R. N. Bryan, and S. M. Resnick, "An image processing system for qualitative and quantitative

volumetric analysis of brain images," *Journal of Computer Assisted Tomography*, vol. 22, no. 5, pp. 827–837, 1998.

[169] F. Kruggel and G. Lohmann, "Automatical adaption of the stereotactical coordinate system in brain MRI datasets," in *the XVth Int. Conf. Inf. Proc. Med. Imag. (IPMI)*. 1997, pp. 471–476, Springer-Verlag.

[170] D. L. Pham, "Robust fuzzy segmentation of magnetic resonance images," in *Proceedings of the Fourteenth IEEE Symposium on Computer-Based Medical Systems (CBMS2001)*, pp. 127–131. IEEE Press, 2001.

[171] D. Lemoine, C. Barillot, B. Gibaud, and E. Pasqualini, "An anatomical-based 3d registration system of multimodality and atlas data in neurosurgery," in *Lecture Notes in Computer Science*, Springer-Verlag, Berlin, 1991, vol. 511.

[172] C. Xu, X. Han, and J. L. Prince, "Improving cortical surface reconstruction accuracy using an anatomically consistent gray matter representation," in *Proc. NeuroImage Hum. Brain Map.*, 2000, vol. 11 of *NeuroImage Suppl.*

[173] A. J. Yezzi Jr. and J. L. Prince, "An evolution pde approach for computing tissue thickness," *IEEE Trans. Med. Imag.*, vol. 22, no. 10, pp. 1332–1339, 2003.

[174] S. M. Resnick, A. F. Goldszal, C. Davatzikos, S. Golski, M. A. Kraut, E. J. Metter, R. N. Bryan, and A. B. Zonderman, "One-year age changes in MRI brain volumes in older adults," *Cerebral Cortex*, vol. 10, no. 5, pp. 464–472, 2000.

[175] A. Cachia, J. F. Mangin, D. Rivière, N. Boddaert, A. Andrade, F. Kherif, P. Sonigo, D. Papadopoulos-Orfanos, M. Zilbovicius, J.-B. Poline, I. Bloch, F. Brunelle, and J. Régis, "A mean curvature based primal sketch to study the cortical folding process from antenatal to adult brain," in *Proc. MICCAI 2001*, W. Niessen and M. Viergever, Eds., Berlin Heidelberg, 2001, LNCS 2208, pp. 897–904, Springer Verlag.

[176] P. Knupp and S. Steinberg, *Fundamentals of Grid Generation*, CRC Press, Boca Raton, FL, 1994.

[177] M. J. Berger and P. Colella, "Local adaptive mesh refinement for shock hydrodynamics," *J. Comput. Phys.*, vol. 82, pp. 64–84, 1984.

[178] B. Milne, *Adaptive Level Set Methods Interfaces*, Ph.D dissertation, Dept. of Math., UC Berkeley, 1995.

[179] M. Sussman, A. S. Almgren, J. B. Bell, P. Colella, L. H. Howell, and M. L. Welcome, "An adaptive level set approach for incompressible two-phase flow," *J. Comput. Phys.*, vol. 148, pp. 81–124, 1999.

[180] M. Droske, B. Meyer, C. Schaller, and M. Rumpf, "An adaptive level set method for medical image segmentation," in *Proc. IPMI 2001*, M. F. Insana and R. M. Leahy, Eds. 2001, LNCS 2082, pp. 416–422, Springer Verlag.

[181] D. Terzopoulos and M. Vasilescu, "Sampling and reconstruction with adaptive meshes," in *Proc. CVPR'91*, Lahaina, HI, 1991, pp. 70–75.

[182] M. Vasilescu and D. Terzopoulos, "Adaptive meshes and shells," in *Proc. CVPR'92*, Champaign, IL, 1992, pp. 829–832.

[183] G. Liao, T. Pan, and J. Shu, "Numerical grid generator based on Moser's deformation method," *Numer. Meth. Part. Diff. Eq.*, vol. 10, pp. 21–31, 1994.

[184] P. Bochev, G. Liao, and G. dela Pena, "Analysis and computation of adaptive moving grids by deformation," *Numer. Meth. Part. Diff. Eq.*, vol. 12, pp. 489–506, 1996.

[185] G. Liao, G. de la Pena, and G. Liao, "A deformation method for moving mesh generation," in *Proc. 8th Intl. Meshing Roundtable*, South Lake Tahoe, CA, 1999, pp. 155–162.

[186] G. Liao, F. Liu, G. de la Pena, D. Peng, and S. Osher, "Level-set-based deformation methods for adaptive grids," *J. Comput. Phys.*, vol. 159, pp. 103–122, 2000.

[187] W. Cao, W. Huang, and R. D. Russell, "A moving mesh method based on the geometric conservation law," *SIAM J. Sci. Comput.*, vol. 24, pp. 118–142, 2002.

[188] C. I. Christov, "Orthogonal coordinate meshes with manageable Jacobian," in *Numerical Grid Generation*, J. F. Thompson, Ed., pp. 885–894. North-Holland, New York, 1982.

[189] M. E. Gurtin, *An Introduction to Continuum Mechanics*, Academic Press, New York, 1981.

[190] W. A. Press, S. A. Teukolsky, W. T. Vetterling, and B. P. Flannery, *Numerical Recipes in C*, Cambridge University Press, New York, NY, 2nd edition, 1995.

[191] E. Braverman, B. Epstein, M. Israeli, and A. Averbuch, "A fast spectral solver for elliptic equations," *J. Sci. Comput.*, vol. 21, pp. 91–128, 2004.

[192] R. C. Buck, *Advanced Calculus*, International Series in Pure and Applied Mathematics. McGraw-Hill, New York, 2nd edition, 1965.

[193] S. A. Ivanenko, "Harmonic mappings," in *Handbook of grid generation*, J. F. Thompson, B. K. Soni, and N. P. Weatherill, Eds., pp. 8:1–43. CRC Press, Boca Raton, 1999.

[194] Y. R. Tsai, L. Cheng, S. Osher, and H. Zhao, "Fast sweeping algorithms for a class of Hamilton-Jacobi equations," Technical Report UCLA-CAM-01-27, Institute for Pure and Applied Mathematics (IPAM), UCLA, 2001.

[195] C. Y. Kao, S. Osher, and Y. R. Tsai, "Fast sweeping methods for a class of static Hamilton-Jacobi equations," Technical Report UCLA-CAM-02-66, Institute for Pure and Applied Mathematics (IPAM), UCLA, 2002.

[196] J. A. Sethian and A. Vladimirsky, "Ordered upwind methods for static Hamilton-Jacobi equations," *Proc. Natl. Acad. Sci.*, vol. 98, no. 20, pp. 11069–11074, 2001.

[197] S. Osher and C. Shu, "Efficient implementation of essentially non-oscillatory shock-capturing schemes, II," *J. Comput. Phys.*, vol. 83, pp. 32–78, 1989.

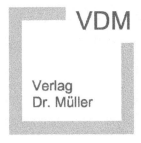

Wissenschaftlicher Buchverlag bietet

kostenfreie

Publikation

von

wissenschaftlichen Arbeiten

Diplomarbeiten, Magisterarbeiten, Master und Bachelor Theses
sowie Dissertationen, Habilitationen und wissenschaftliche Monographien

Sie verfügen über eine wissenschaftliche Abschlußarbeit zu aktuellen oder zeitlosen
Fragestellungen, die hohen inhaltlichen und formalen Ansprüchen genügt,
und haben **Interesse an einer honorarvergüteten Publikation**?

Dann senden Sie bitte erste Informationen über Ihre Arbeit per Email
an info@vdm-verlag.de. Unser Außenlektorat meldet sich umgehend bei Ihnen.

VDM Verlag Dr. Müller Aktiengesellschaft & Co. KG
Dudweiler Landstraße 125a
D - 66123 Saarbrücken

www.vdm-verlag.de

www.ingramcontent.com/pod-product-compliance
Lightning Source LLC
La Vergne TN
LVHW022308060326
832902LV00020B/3349